TRANSPLANTATION

Other titles in the *New Clinical Applications* Series:

Dermatology (Series Editor Dr J. L. Verbov)
Dermatological Surgery
Superficial Fungal Infections
Talking Points in Dermatology – I
Treatment in Dermatology
Current Concepts in Contact Dermatitis
Talking Points in Dermatology – II
Tumours, Lymphomas and Selected Paraproteinaemias
Relationships in Dermatology
Talking Points in Dermatology – III
Mycobacterial Skin Diseases

Cardiology (Series Editor Dr D. Longmore)
Cardiology Screening

Rheumatology (Series Editors Dr J. J. Calabro and Dr W. Carson Dick)
Ankylosing Spondylitis
Infections and Arthritis
Osteoporosis

Nephrology (Series Editor Professor G. R. D. Catto)
Continuous Ambulatory Peritoneal Dialysis
Management of Renal Hypertension
Chronic Renal Failure
Calculus Disease
Pregnancy and Renal Disorders
Multisystem Diseases
Glomerulonephritis I
Glomerulonephritis II
Haemodialysis
Urinary Tract Infections

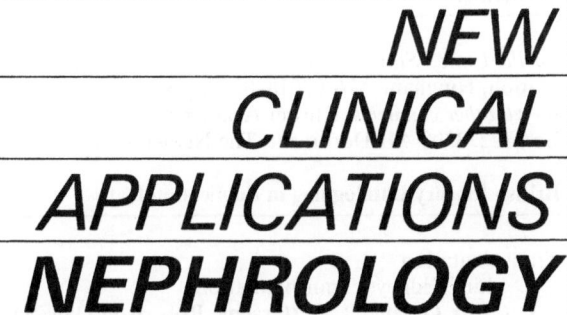

NEW
CLINICAL
APPLICATIONS
NEPHROLOGY

TRANSPLANTATION

Editor

G. R. D. CATTO

MD, DSc, FRCP (Lond., Edin. and Glas.)

Professor of Medicine and Therapeutics
University of Aberdeen
UK

WKAP ARCHIEF

KLUWER ACADEMIC PUBLISHERS
DORDRECHT / BOSTON / LONDON

Distributors

for the United States and Canada: Kluwer Academic Publishers, PO Box 358, Accord Station, Hingham, MA 02018–0358, USA
for all other countries: Kluwer Academic Publishers Group, Distribution Center, PO Box 322, 3300 AH Dordrecht, The Netherlands

British Library Cataloguing in Publication Data

Transplantation
  1. Man. Kidneys. Transplantation
  I. Catto, Graeme R. D. (Graeme Robertson Dawson),
  1945– II. Series
  617'.4610592

  ISBN-13: 978-94-010-6872-7   e-ISBN-13: 978-94-009-0855-0
  DOI: 10.1007/978-94-009-0855-0

Copyright

CONTENTS

LIST OF AUTHORS

R. Y. Calne
Department of Surgery,
University of Cambridge,
Addenbrooke's Hospital,
Hills Road,
Cambridge CB2 2QQ
UK

J. R. Chapman
Renal Unit,
Westmead Hospital,
Westmead,
Sydney,
NSW 2145
Australia
and
Tissue Typing Laboratory,
Red Cross Blood Transfusion
Service,
153 Clarence Street,
Sydney,
NSW 2000
Australia

P. Friend
Department of Surgery,
University of Cambridge,
Addenbrooke's Hospital,
Hills Road,
Cambridge CB2 2QQ
UK

V. C. Joysey
Tissue Typing Laboratory
Addenbrooke's Hospital,
Hills Road,
Cambridge CB2 2QQ
UK

A. I. Lazarovits
John P. Robarts Research Institute.
University Hospital,
339 Windermere Road,
London,
Ontario N6A 5A5
Canada

C. R. Stiller
John P. Robarts Research Institute
University Hospital,
339 Windermere Road,
London,
Ontario N6A 5A5
Canada

A. Ting
Nuffield Department of Surgery,
John Radcliffe Hospital,
Headington,
Oxford OX3 9DU
UK

D. J. G. White
Department of Surgery,
University of Cambridge,
Addenbrooke's Hospital,
Hills Road,
Cambridge CB2 2QQ
UK

SERIES EDITOR'S FOREWORD

Renal transplantation is now accepted as the treatment of choice for patients with end-stage renal failure. During the last decade both patients and graft survival rates have increased significantly and when assessed at one year are now greater than 90% and 80% respectively. These marked improvements have occurred at a time when increasing numbers of patients in the older age groups and with more complex forms of renal disease are being accepted for transplantation. The reasons for the improved clinical results are not fully understood but are probably linked with changes in blood transfusion policy, tissue typing policy and drug therapy.

These topics, together with immunological monitoring and details of how to treat the highly sensitized patient, are fully covered in this volume. All the chapters have been written by recognized experts in their field. Not only are the recent advances well documented but the likely future developments in management are identified and discussed. As renal transplantation is now the single most common form of treatment for renal failure, the information presented in this volume should prove of value to all with an interest in current clinical practice.

ABOUT THE EDITOR

Professor Graeme R. D. Catto is Professor in Medicine and Therapeutics at the University of Aberdeen and Honorary Consultant Physician/Nephrologist to the Grampian Health Board. His current interest in transplant immunology was stimulated as a Harkness Fellow at Harvard Medical School and the Peter Bent Brighton Hospital, Boston, USA. He is a member of many medical societies including the Association of Physicians of Great Britain and Ireland, the Renal Association and the Transplantation Society. He has published widely on transplant and reproductive immunology, calcium metabolism and general nephrology.

1
BLOOD TRANSFUSION POLICY

J. R. CHAPMAN

INTRODUCTION

Transfusion of blood into patients awaiting renal transplantation did not require policy decisions during the early phase of the history of transplantation in the 1960s. Instead, blood transfusion was a clinical requirement for the successful dialysis of uraemic patients. Blood transfusion in the late 1980s and the 1990s has, by contrast, become a less frequently mandated therapy with the advent of efficient low-volume dialysers, reduced blood loss, alternative blood volume expanders and, finally, with erythropoietin. The hazards of blood transfusion have also, during those 20 years, become better appreciated. Every renal physician must therefore now have a policy on blood transfusion, particularly for those patients who are awaiting either · a cadaver or a living related kidney transplant. The span of 20 years of research and clinical experience has provided an enormous literature from which it is possible to find reference to the therapeutic advantage of almost any policy on blood transfusion. In this chapter, I will attempt to pick my way through that literature to highlight some of the evidence used to support the various current policies on blood transfusion. The issues could have subsided into a consensus clinical practice but for the problem of viral transmission by blood and recent evidence that the 'transfusion effect' in clinical transplantation may be waning.

RAISING THE ISSUE

Pre-existing humoral sensitization of patients to human leukocyte antigens was recognized as associated with catastrophic loss of a renal allograft in 1965[1]. It had long been recognized that antibodies to those antigens could be raised by multiple transfusions of blood since Dausset first demonstrated leuko-agglutinating antibodies in that situation[2]. It was thus thought that blood transfusion would be a disadvantage to prospective recipients of renal transplants. The firm evidence from Patel and Terasaki's work on the lymphocytotoxic crossmatch, published in 1969[3], dispelled any doubt from the majority of physicians' minds that the only policy to maintain on blood transfusion was avoidance. There were four clinical papers in the 1960s which cast small clouds of doubt over the security of the clear cut antithesis to blood evident in the early 1970s. Michielsen[4] and Dossetor et al.[5] both commented on the fact that patients transfused with blood appeared stubbornly to contradict the immunology theorists by frequently undergoing renal transplantation successfully. In a widely unquoted paper in an Australian journal, Morris et al. studied 43 primary cadaver graft recipients and noted no correlation between the grade of rejection and number of transfusions[6]. They postulated that multiple blood transfusions might lead to a state of partial tolerance of the graft, in an analogous way to the known effect of donor antigen pretreatment in animal models of transplantation. The founding pioneer of clinical transplantation, David Hume, also commented upon the disparity between practice and theory with regard to blood transfusion[7].

It perhaps should not have come as an immense surprise when data were presented showing that blood transfusion actually improved the outcome of renal transplantation. The paper by Opelz and his colleagues, presented at the 4th Congress of the Transplantation Society in 1972[8], showed that one-year graft survival was 29% in untransfused patients, 43% in those given between one and ten units of blood, and 66% in those given more than ten units. Scepticism has been the word most frequently used to describe the thoughts of those hearing that evidence. 'Scepticism' bred thousands of research studies, spent millions of dollars and pounds, stimulated interest in the field of transplantation, and probably contributed eventually to a con-

2

siderable improvement in the outcome of renal transplantation. It was somewhat ironic to hear the same speaker present evidence to the 11th Congress of the Transplantation Society, which suggested that in the mid-1980s, the effect of transfusion may no longer be discerned in current clinical practice[9].

CLINICAL EXPERIENCE

In the early 1980s it was possible for authoritative speakers to state[10] 'virtually everybody agrees that pretransplant blood transfusion will improve graft survival'. The evidence supporting the 'transfusion effect' has come from controlled and uncontrolled single-centre trials and multicentre studies. In Figure 1.1, the changes in graft survival at one year between those patients who had not received blood and those transfused varying numbers and varying preparations of blood are compared by the year of publication of the paper. Many trials of transfusion are not recorded here because of lack of appropriate data for comparison, but this figure represents a reasonable sample of the clinical experience. A number of generalizations can be gleaned from reading these 47 papers. Firstly, the majority of randomized and controlled data was collected during the mid-1970s and published in 1977 and 1978. Secondly, studies which failed to demonstrate a significant effect of transfusion can be discerned as having one of three exceptions to the general experience: small numbers of patients; high survival rates of untransfused patients; or worse than usual survival of transfused patients. Thirdly, the survival of untransfused recipients has tended to improve over the years. The blood transfusion effect may thus be taken as an established fact in patients transplanted using azathioprine and corticosteroids. Clinical application of the message of these studies was demonstrated by a progressive fall in the percentage of untransfused patients receiving a renal transplant. In 1975, 35% of all patients were untransfused, a figure which fell to 19% by 1980, and 4% by 1983[11]. There has been a slow reversal of that trend visible in data from the Collaborative Transplant Study in patients treated with cyclosporin, 9% being untransfused in 1984, 8% in 1985 and 13% in 1986[12]. Deliberate blood transfusion policies have been largely responsible for these changing figures.

3

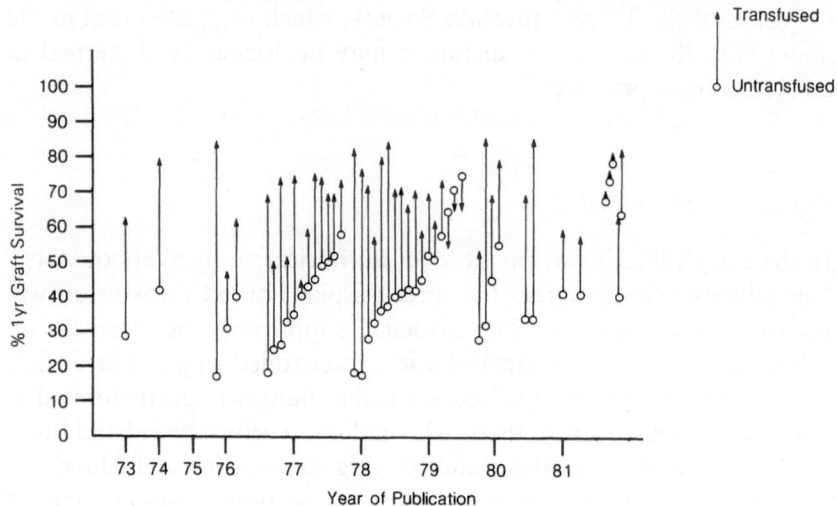

FIGURE 1.1 First cadaver allograft survival in recipients who were untransfused compared with those who had been transfused one or more units of blood, reported in 47 different studies. The studies have been arranged by year of publication of the paper. The five most recent studies were published in 1986 and 1987

Questions about the transfusion effect rather than questioning the existence of the effect thus became the most pressing issues in both clinical and experimental transplantation. The benefit derived from blood transfusion, it was argued, should surely hold the key to tolerance of an allograft and thus unlock the door to a truly successful mode of therapy.

Which blood product, how much, how frequently, when, in which patients? Is the mechanism mediated through selection of donor–recipient pairs, selection of responder status, induction of enhancing antibodies, induction of anti-idiotypic antibodies, or induction of suppressor cells? What are the disadvantages, how can they be avoided? Many of these questions can only be given equivocal answers despite the effort devoted to unravelling the problem.

4

Which blood product?

Transfusion of blood leads to development of antibodies to human leukocyte antigens (HLA). Thus, a constant theme running through the debates on blood transfusion is the disadvantage of stimulating lymphocytotoxic antibodies, which subsequently make transplantation of a negative crossmatch kidney difficult or impossible in a number of patients. I discuss the problem of sensitization in more detail below, but this serious consequence of a deliberate transfusion policy led to numerous attempts to provide a blood product which would both improve allograft survival rates and avoid humoral sensitization.

The initial data on the transfusion effect were largely gleaned from observation of clinical practice where the commonest preparation has been 'packed cells'. Both whole blood and packed cells have consistently caused improvement in graft survival. Data from the UCLA transplant registry have, for example, repeatedly shown an equivalent benefit for these two preparations[13,14]. In the earlier reports, washed blood did not, however, appear to yield such a strong effect and frozen–thawed blood produced no benefit[13,15]. The careful study from Leiden[15] for example, showed an 80% graft survival in those transfused with just one unit of washed cells (i.e. a leukocyte-poor preparation), while a total of between one and three units of frozen–thawed blood (which was regarded as leukocyte-free) was associated with 33% graft survival. A discordant view has come from Boston where frozen blood reduced the incidence of humoral sensitization but did not alter graft survival rates when compared with whole blood[16]. The explanation for these divergent views on the use of frozen blood may lie in the method of storage since the 'agglomerating' technique of Huggins in Boston preserved more leukocytes than the conventional centrifugation and washing technique. The trend towards use of frozen blood has not been widely perpetuated, while washed blood and more recently (and perhaps more effectively) filtered blood have been used, in the context of clinical necessity rather than deliberate transfusion policy, in an attempt to reduce the rate of sensitization.

The concept that platelet transfusion would not lead to humoral sensitization but would modify subsequent immune responses beneficially was espoused by Batchelor *et al*[17]. Platelets are known to adsorb soluble HLA class I antigens into their surface, but do not carry class II antigens. Successful allograft tolerance has been reported in a number of small animal models in which donor class I antigens have been transfused and it was thus of interest when a beneficial effect of platelet transfusion was published from the primate centre in the Netherlands[18]. Rhesus monkeys had been transfused with purified platelets and then transplanted with a kidney from a third monkey. None of the platelet-transfused, but most of the blood-transfused control animals, developed cytotoxic antibodies. More importantly, renal transplant outcome of the platelet transfused animals was particularly good. Supportive evidence was forthcoming from the primate centre in Atlanta[19] and in the mongrel dog[20] but not beagle dog models[21]. It was felt that the general conclusions from these animal studies warranted pilot studies in the clinical situation. Three trials have now reported mildly conflicting data on the benefits of platelet transfusions[22–24]. In the Oxford study[22], it was shown that minor contamination of the platelet preparation by leukocytes (15×10^6) resulted in a high degree of sensitization (42% developing cytotoxic antibodies after three transfusions) while a pure preparation of platelets, with less than 5×10^6 leukocytes per transfusion, did not sensitize. Graft survival rates were, however, unexpectedly bad leading to curtailment of the study. The Spanish experience[23] was similar, in that graft survival was not improved by platelets, but the French trial[24] yielded both low sensitization rates and good early allograft survival from a pure preparation. Platelet transfusion, while conceptually attractive, has thus not generally borne out in clinical practice the promise of animal models, and is no longer being actively pursued as an alternative to whole blood or packed cells.

Whole blood, packed cells and frozen–thawed blood with preserved leukocytes all evoke the 'transfusion effect' while platelets probably do not. The leukocyte component, therefore, may be the significant fraction required to achieve improved transplant outcome. If this is true, transfusion of buffy coat layers would be expected to emulate whole blood. Norman and his colleagues[25] transfused buffy coat pooled from five or ten donors and showed significant improvement in renal allograft survival from the larger dosage, thus confirming the efficacy of buffy coat. Supporting data have been supplied from a

Japanese study of donor-specific buffy coat transfusion in single haplotype-matched, living related transplants[26]. Inclusion of leukocytes in the blood product thus seems a desirable and possibly necessary feature of a transfusion policy designed to improve allograft outcome.

How much blood?

A few microlitres of infected blood are sufficient to transmit hepatitis or human immunodeficiency viruses. Aliquots of 20 ml of blood given in repeated doses are able to stimulate production of antibodies to HLA antigens in volunteers[27], but the volume required to produce the transfusion effect in renal transplantation is less easily settled.

An effect of dose was reported in the initial paper[8] in 1973, where patients given more than ten units fared better than those given between one and ten units, who, in their turn, had better graft survival rates than untransfused patients. The UCLA registry data has continued to show a dose effect up to 1983, with those given between one and four units having a graft survival rate at one year that was intermediate between the untransfused patient and those given five to twenty units[14]. Graft survival in the polytransfused patient (20 units or more) reported to the International registries has usually been reported as worse than those given fewer units of blood. This has been attributed to the bias introduced by patients who are at a high risk of medical complications being clustered into the polytransfused group[11]. Results from the two large registries are detailed in Table 1.1, from which it can be seen that there is a significant effect from transfusion of a single unit of blood. Graft survival does appear to increase with the number of units given, though the increased benefit per unit is quite small after 5 units. The risks of infection and sensitization are, on the other hand, either constant or increase with each unit given. Single-centre studies of relatively small numbers of patients have demonstrated that one unit of blood is sufficient to produce a significant transfusion effect[15], but those studies do not rule out further benefit from subsequent units.

The majority of transfusion protocols have settled on elective donations of between three and five units of blood before a transplant

7

TABLE 1.1   One-year graft survival related to the number of units of blood transfused before transplantation

Reference	No. of Units transfused	1-year graft survival (%)
ULCA Registry (1985)[14]	0	44
	1–4	59
	5–20	64
	20	52–65
CTS (1983)[11]	0	43
	1	58
	2–4	66
	5–10	69
	11–20	72
	20	63

is performed. There is no substantial evidence which distinguishes between these choices on the basis of transplant outcome and so the decision must be based upon factors such as convenience, availability, and risks of transfusing increasing units of blood.

Fresh or stored blood?

There is very little data on the relative effects of fresh and stored whole blood or packed cells, though it is known that viable leukocyte numbers decline with storage time. It is possible that fresh blood (less than 3 days old) stimulates a more efficient humoral response than blood 10–14 days old, but it is not known which features are important for obtaining improved allograft outcome. There is one study that suggests that fresh blood is better than stored blood for inducing the transfusion effect[28] but the issue has not been widely explored.

When to transfuse?

Blood may be given at the time of operation or many years before the patient develops renal failure and requires transplantation. There are data to support the efficacy of both these intervals between transfusion and operation. Transfusion at the time of the operation has the advantage that the blood will not lead to humoral sensitization, thereby precluding the transplant with a positive crossmatch. Stiller was the first to suggest, on the basis of a retrospective analysis of his data, that there was a beneficial effect of preoperative blood transfusion in previously untransfused patients[29]. He received criticism for his paper but others were sufficiently interested to examine their own data and establish a prospective randomized controlled trial of the effect of two units of peroperative blood[30]. In that trial, graft survival at one year was 85% in the transfused group and 34% in the untransfused control group, thus demonstrating a significant effect of blood given at operation. The extreme effect shown in the single-centre trial has not been confirmed in the uncontrolled registry data, which have, however, demonstrated a small benefit from peroperative transfusion in previously untransfused patients (5% increase in one-year graft survival)[14]. Data from the South-Eastern Organ Procurement Foundation (SEOPF) have also supported the view that perioperative transfusion (which they defined as given at the time of, or within ten days before the transplant) conferred benefits[31]. Graft survival increased from 41% to 49% at one year when perioperative blood was given to those patients not previously transfused. An advantage for perioperative blood in patients who had already been transfused could, however, only be demonstrated in sensitized recipients receiving a regraft.

The general experience has been that while peroperative and perioperative blood may confer measurable benefit, deliberate transfusion protocols given well before transplantation produce a greater effect. Interesting data were obtained from the UCLA registry by examining graft survival in patients given just one unit of blood at different intervals before transplantation[14]. The greatest improvement in graft survival was achieved in patients transfused between one day and one week preoperatively. A further slight benefit could be observed by waiting two to three months after transfusion before transplantation, but the effects were still clearly evident in those transfused two or more years previously. The authors of that study have also stated that the same persistence of the transfusion effect was evident in multiply transfused patients. A variety of authors have supported a variety of specific 'time frames' within which transfusion and transplantation produce optimal results. The practical aspects of even attempting to achieve those intervals are not possible for almost all cadaver allograft programmes. It is therefore reassuring to be able to fall back upon the data surrounding the concept of any interval longer than a few weeks. Most programmes would also want to allow two to four weeks following transfusion for development of anti-HLA antibodies to occur before placing the patient on an active transplant waiting list. One question, that has yet to be resolved, is whether or not one should retransfuse patients whose previous transfusions were many years ago. To a certain extent this debate centres on the philosophy of whether or not it is wise to let sleeping dogs lie, rather than on secure data.

Transfusing the donor

While transfusion of blood to the donor of bone marrow might be expected to alter the outcome of a bone marrow graft, it would perhaps not be expected to have a significant effect on a solid organ allograft. There are, however, animal data which suggest that transfusion of third-party blood, containing viable leukocytes, two days before nephrectomy and transplantation improves the outcome in transfused recipients[32]. One retrospective study from three Scandinavian centres has suggested that the same phenomenon could be observed in clinical practice, with improved graft survival of kidneys from donors transfused within two days of nephrectomy[33,34]. More recent data have been presented showing that a similar benefit may be derived from using kidneys from trauma deaths[35]. Whether it is a donor blood transfusion effect or the physiological nature of kidneys from young male trauma deaths that explains these findings, they are inextricably bound pending a controlled trial of blood transfusion before nephrectomy. While awaiting that trial, transplant units will continue to accept as many cadaveric organs as possible, irrespective of transfusion or trauma without the complication of elective donor transfusion.

DISADVANTAGES OF BLOOD TRANSFUSION

Viral infection

The first recipient of a renal allograft performed in 1933 almost certainly died as a result of an incompatible blood transfusion[36]. The general hazards of transfusing blood apply as much to renal transplant recipients as to any other patient. Though it is beyond the scope of this chapter to describe these in detail, it is impossible to ignore the occasionally fatal consequences of taking blood from one person and giving it to another. Two particular hazards do need comment, namely hepatitis and human immunodeficiency viruses. Hepatitis B swept through renal units causing many patient and staff deaths in the 1960s, since when renal physicians and staff of dialysis units have had a particular regard for blood-borne virus infection. It is, of course, routine practice to identify and exclude hepatitis B virus from transfused blood, but exclusion of non-A, non-B hepatitis remains an unrealized goal. The history of unknowing transfer of human immunodeficiency virus (HIV) by blood transfusion is familiar to all. Transfer of the virus by renal transplantation has also been reported with devastating consequences for the recipients[37]. It has become clear that presence of antibodies to HIV constitutes an absolute barrier to transplantation, at present, because of the devastatingly rapid progression to symptomatic disease and death produced by the addition of immunosuppressive medication. The smallest risk of HIV transmission is thus a major consideration in transfusion policies and it is clear why constant re-evaluation of the benefits of transfusion must be undertaken by those practising medicine where HIV is most prevalent[38].

Sensitization

The major common disadvantage of transfusing blood into potential renal allograft recipients is development of antibodies to HLA class I molecules. This disadvantage was the rationale for avoiding transfusion and the fact of overall advantage does not reduce the huge disadvantages conferred upon a minority of patients by transfusion of blood.

11

Dausset and his colleagues demonstrated in 1954 the role of multiple blood transfusions in production of leukoagglutinating antibodies[39], and postulated that they might be directed against either single or multiple antigens. It was subsequently shown that between 9 and 26 weekly injections of 20 ml of blood are required to stimulate a primary response, but that even 66 weekly injections failed to elicit a response in one person[27]. By contrast, only two or three injections stimulated a secondary response. In the dialysis population, sensitization by whole blood or packed cells is also dose dependent, as shown by a study of 550 patients where 4% were 'highly sensitized' after five transfusions, 7% after ten, and 12% after 20[40]. Multiparous women constitute the major group at risk since male and nulliparous patients, though they become sensitized, rarely become highly sensitized by blood transfusion. In an extensive examination of the role of sensitization in 737 patients reported to the UCLA transplant registry, less than 2% of males developed cytotoxic antibodies to more than 90% of a random panel despite 10 units of blood[41]. In female patients, by contrast, the rate of high sensitization ($\geqslant$90% PRA) was 14%, representing a seven-fold increased risk. The predominant cause of this extra risk was shown to be pregnancy, since nulliparous females had an equivalent risk to males, while those who had either one to three, or more than three pregnancies, were at considerable risk of becoming highly sensitized (approximately 18% and 30% respectively). Lower overall rates of sensitization have been seen in prospective studies but the pattern of risks has been confirmed by a number of studies. Parous women can be distinguished by their ability to develop lymphocytotoxic antibodies after as few as one unit of blood, multiparity and multiple transfusions together leading to a very significant risk of becoming untransplantable. Highly sensitized males, on the other hand, have almost always rejected a previous transplant, transfusion alone being insufficient. Scornik et al. have used flow cytometric techniques to demonstrate low levels of antibodies (undetected by cytotoxicity tests) directed at lymphocytes in parous women who develop high levels of lymphocytotoxic antibodies after blood transfusion[42]. They have suggested that elective transfusion should be restricted to patients in whom no antibodies can be detected by the flow cytometer and have provided some evidence that this policy reduces the rate of sensitization[43].

12

An alternative approach is to define the blood product which yields the lowest rate of sensitization while preserving the transfusion effect. I have already discussed a number of studies designed to minimize lymphocytotoxic antibody formation. Single-centre studies have, for example, demonstrated low levels of sensitization from frozen–thawed blood[16], pure platelets[22] and buffy coat[25]. The multicentre SEOPF experience between 1977 and 1982, on the other hand, showed very little difference between sensitization rates of whole blood, packed cells, frozen blood and washed blood[44]. The only significant effect was seen when comparing the sensitization rates of whole blood and frozen or washed blood given to regraft recipients. Filtration of blood through the current generation of efficient filters may reduce the rate of sensitization experienced from filtered as opposed to washed blood, but my data suggest that the total number of leukocytes will have to be less than 5×10^6 per transfusion. This level cannot be approached in routine clinical practice[22].

If it not possible reliably to avoid the patient at risk and it is not possible to use a non-sensitizing blood product, then perhaps it will prove possible to suppress the immune response of the patient. One small trial of azathioprine in patients given third-party blood transfusions does not encourage belief in the efficacy of this approach since more of the azathioprine-treated patients became sensitized than the controls[45].

Since we are unable to predict the patient, choose the blood product or modify the patient's response, we must, in desperation, turn the argument around and suggest that sensitization does not matter[46], or is a laudable result of transfusion[47]. This argument centres on the concept that a patient who becomes highly sensitized for a brief period has henceforth to receive a kidney that has a negative crossmatch with serum samples taken at the time of peak sensitization. A proportion of patients treated by Cardella et al. were given repeated blood transfusions after becoming sensitized and lost their antibodies[46]. These patients were subsequently transplanted with a kidney from a donor who had a positive crossmatch using serum from the period of peak sensitization but negative with serum taken at the time of the transplant. The success of these grafts demonstrated that, at least in this group of patients, the high level of sensitization did not seem to confer a lasting disadvantage. Norman et al.[47] among others[48], have published data showing improved graft survival in patients who developed more than 20% reactivity to lymphocyte panels – despite transplantation across a positive crossmatch with the peak reactive samples. The majority of patients who develop lymphocytotoxic antibodies after transfusion lose them within nine months if they are not transfused again and some lose them even if they are transfused. The solution to the dilemma of sensitization from elective transfusion would therefore appear to be the healing virtues of the passage of time. It is, however, worth sounding a note of caution since multiparous women who become highly sensitized following blood transfusion can have lymphocytotoxic antibodies which persist for many years and not all transplants performed across a peak positive crossmatch result are successful[49].

Transfusion after graft failure

The majority of patients with lasting broadly reactive lymphocytotoxic antibodies have become sensitized either during or soon after primary allograft rejection. The solution to the problem that these patients pose across the world has centred on prevention, firstly by reducing acute allograft rejection in most primary cadaver allograft recipients, and secondly by improving matching for HLA class I antigens[50]. The role of blood transfusion given during the course of the initial unsuccessful transplant has been difficult to dissect. In my data[51], two thirds of patients who became highly sensitized following graft failure were sensitized before graft nephrectomy but one third developed their antibodies after nephrectomy. In the latter group of 24 patients, 15 received blood during or soon after the operation and became highly sensitized after nephrectomy, while 9 were not sensitized after nephrectomy but became highly sensitized following blood transfusions given during the subsequent weeks or months. Scornik has also reported this phenomenon and has demonstrated that, while cytotoxic antibodies only appeared after blood transfusion, the antigen specificity was carried by the graft and not the blood[52]. Blood transfusion, either during or after graft rejection, may thus act as a non-specific stimulus to lymphocytotoxic antibody production.

RECENT EXPERIENCE WITH ELECTIVE TRANSFUSIONS

Cyclosporine has improved overall allograft survival rates wherever it has been used. The efficacy of this drug has led some authors to suggest that its use has altered the ground rules of transplantation. Formal re-examination of the effect of HLA antigen matching did not require a change in policy, since transplantation continues across all grades of tissue antigen match. Re-examination of the role of blood transfusion, by contrast, has required the abandonment of the elective transfusion policies which were instigated on the secure evidence of the 1970s. Scandia Transplant took this decision and suspended elective transfusion of prospective transplant recipients in November 1982[53]. No effect on graft survival of either matching for HLA or blood transfusion could be shown at one or two years.

This authoritative study from a highly regarded group was based on 147 untransfused and 334 transfused patients and created a ripple in the previously calm acceptance of elective transfusions. Three points need to be made about this study before its message can be universally applied. Firstly the overall graft and patient survival rates were disappointing (68% of grafts and 89% of patients surviving the first year). Secondly, there was a significant effect for HLA-B and DR matching on the frequency of acute rejections which one might expect to be translated to differences in graft survival if sufficient patients are followed for long enough. Thirdly, untransfused patients were not allocated to transfused and non-transfused groups, but were compared with patients who happened to have been transfused. It is, therefore, wrong to ascribe to this study the virtues of a randomized controlled trial, since there were definite and measurable differences other than blood transfusion between these groups.

Criticisms aside, this was clearly an important study and the issue was selected for debate at the 11th Transplantation Society Congress. Opelz[54] and Groth[55] were expected to debate the issue and conclude that Scandia Transplant experience did not mirror the rest of the world. The debate was, however, enlivened by Opelz's presentation of the Collaborative Transplant Study (CTS) data which, far from disagreeing, was actually in concordance with Scandia Transplant. The transfusion effect appeared to have vanished in 1986. One hundred and twenty-eight untransfused patients transplanted in 1982 and 1983 using cyclosporine who were reported to the CTS, did indeed have worse graft survivals than 1486 transfused patients. By contrast, 452 untransfused cyclosporine-treated patients who were transplanted in 1984 and 1985 did not fare much worse than 5451 transfused patients, in terms of actuarial graft survival at one year. Experienced use of cyclosporine could not, however, be regarded as the explanation for this observed effect because the same improvement occurred in graft survival of untransfused azathioprine-treated patients. The transfusion effect disappeared from the CTS data because of progressively improved survival of untransfused patients, rather than deterioration in the outcome of transfused patients.

This study was not randomized or controlled and there are many potential biases introduced by the nature of this international survey. The data have, however, been largely confirmed by a further CTS analysis of patients transplanted in 1986[12], in whom only about a 5% difference in graft survival rates at one year is seen between transfused and untransfused patients. The UCLA registry data agree that there has been a progressive rise in graft survival rates in untransfused patients, but disagree with the CTS by still finding a benefit from transfusion[56]. Evidence that also conflicts with the CTS analysis has come from the San Francisco Transplant Service, where untransfused recipients transplanted between 1983 and 1985 fared worse than transfused patients[38]. The solution of this conflict will not be easily achieved, largely because the factors which improved graft survival in transfused patients have never been satisfactorily elucidated. Despite more than 15 years of research effort, we are still observing a phenomenon, as opposed to manipulating the immune response selectively.

Opelz's own response to the CTS and Scandia Transplant results was to urge caution[54]. I agree that wholesale abandonment of blood transfusion protocols would be unwise for several reasons. Firstly, the data may appear secure, but that does not imply that the conclusions are applicable to all units. Secondly, the measure of outcome that has been analysed so far is the difference in one-year graft survival between transfused and untransfused patients. Success at one year is clearly important, but success at ten or twenty years must be the aim of most transplant programmes. A small or insignificant effect at one year may be a major effect at the five-year mark or beyond. One year is thus, in my view, too early to abandon a policy that has much clinical experience and many randomized controlled trials to support it. The data do, however, once more justify randomization of untransfused patients to transfusion protocols or control groups, and these trials will no doubt follow.

DONOR-SPECIFIC TRANSFUSIONS

Graft survival of one haplotype-matched living related grafts with a high mixed lymphocyte culture (MLC) index was not better than could be achieved with cadaveric transplantation. By contrast, HLA-identical sibling grafts and single haplotype-matched grafts with a low MLC index did fare better than cadaver grafts. Random blood transfusion of recipients of mismatched living related grafts had been seen to improve outcome and so, following the lead of Newton and Anderson[57], Salvatierra and his colleagues embarked upon a policy of transfusion of three units of fresh blood from the prospective kidney donor to the recipient[58]. Development of antibodies to donor T lymphocytes was seen in 29% of the first 45 patients studied, thus excluding transplantation in a significant minority of patients. Graft survival in the remaining patients after transplantation was, however, better than anticipated, with a low incidence of acute rejection episodes and failure of only one graft (due to stopping immunosuppression). The donor-specific effect of blood was well known in animal models but this was the first convincing demonstration of the effect in clinical practice. Salvatierra et al. postulated two mechanisms by which the good results of transplantation were achieved by donor specific transfusion (DST). Firstly, the segregation of 'responders' from 'non-responders', with the latter expected to do well; and secondly, modification of the recipient's immune response. Evidence against the 'selection theory' to explain the DST effect was that third-party blood could also be shown to have an effect, and that a small proportion of patients had early and abrupt rejection episodes but went on to have successful grafts.

Donor-specific transfusion was subsequently investigated by other groups who, in general, confirmed the San Francisco message. DST was an effective method of improving graft survival in mismatched living related transplantation. The problem of humoral sensitization as a result of DST was regarded in two different lights. One argument proposed that sensitization was a clear demonstration of alloreactivity to the donor and that the graft would have been likely to be rejected; sensitization was therefore a useful evil. The second view was that sensitization was an unnecessary phenomenon of no relevance to transplant outcome, and therefore should be suppressed. Glass and his colleagues compared two consecutive DST protocols which addressed this issue[59]. Sensitization in 36 patients given DST together with azathioprine was 11% compared with 27% of 56 patients given DST alone. Graft survival was unaffected and it was thought that the azathioprine protocol was of value because of the lower rate of sensitization. The concept that DST was only applicable to one haplotype disparate pairs with high MLC indices of reactivity was abandoned in this study, and DST was given not only to living related but also to unrelated donors. The issue of limiting sensitization by azathioprine has subsequently been subjected to more critical analysis[60]. It has become apparent that patients who were unsensitized at the start of the DST protocol had a moderate risk (19%) of developing transient antibodies which could be reduced to 6% by azathioprine. Sensitized patients with antibodies reactive against more than 10% of a random panel, on the other hand, had a high risk (56%) of developing broadly reactive and persistent antibodies which were not significantly reduced by azathioprine. These data are consistent with those from Columbus, Ohio where multiparous women and patients who had rejected a previous graft were at the greatest risk of sensitization[61]. It was therefore suggested that DST might be better avoided in those patients at high risk of becoming sensitized.

'Sensitization' is a general term describing development of cytotoxic antibodies after DST. It is, however, possible to classify the antibodies by target cell (B or T lymphocyte) or antigen specificity (autoreactive, anti-HLA class I or class II). A transplant against a positive cell T cell crossmatch, which developed after DST, was reported to be hyperacutely rejected[62], and there has been a considerable reluctance to transplant against an antibody that is assumed to be directed at a donor HLA class I mismatched antigen. Transient or persistent positive crossmatches with B lymphocytes do not have that feared reputation and many successful transplants have been performed. Salvatierra et al. have used a flow cytometer crossmatch to distinguish

18

positive B cell crossmatches due to weak anti-HLA class I antibodies from those specific for B cells and presumed to be directed at class II antigens[62]. They reported transplantation in 45 patients with a positive cytotoxic B cell crossmatch but negative T cell cytotoxic and flow cytometer crossmatches; only two grafts failed (4%). One study has addressed the problem of transplanting patients despite a peak positive T cell crossmatch which was rendered negative by plasmapheresis in four patients[63]. Two of the patients suffered severe rejections requiring dialysis but all four grafts were functioning between six months and two years after transplantation. It was clearly possible to achieve successful transplantation in this group's experience, but it was equally clear that it was a procedure that one might only turn to as a last resort. Two of the four patients transplanted after natural disappearance of their antibodies lost their grafts, the remaining two having well functioning grafts beyond one year. Before transplanting in this situation, one might wish to know whether the two outcomes can be separated by closer analysis of the cause of the peak serum positive crossmatch.

The same process of blood product selection has been applied to donor-specific transfusion as I described for random transfusions. Three units of fresh whole blood were used in the initial protocol[58], but there are advocates of stored blood[64]; buffy coat[63]; a combination of fresh and stored blood in 100 ml aliquots[65]; and two, instead of three, units[66]. All of these protocols appear to work and it would be hard to choose between them on a scientific basis. There has been no enthusiasm for donor-specific transfusion of pure red cell or platelet preparations, since there is a belief that the leukocyte fraction is relevant.

The advantages of DST seem to be perpetuated in the medium- to long-term data[62], though there has been doubt cast on the efficacy of DST in patients treated with cyclosporin[67,68]. The paper from Kahan's group[67] could have been reporting the effect of random blood transfusion in single haplotype-matched transplants, had they chosen to interpret their data in that way. The suggestion that random blood may be as good as donor-specific blood, at least in patients transplanted using cyclosporin, has been made on the basis of data reported to the CTS[12,69]. The UCLA registry provided further support for equal efficacy of DST and random blood in matched and single haplotype

19

matched living relative transplantation[70]. The Scandinavian study[68], however, echoed the nihilism of their results of transfusion in cadaveric transplantation by suggesting that only panel reactive antibody status had any influence on the outcome of single haplotype matched living related transplants. These observations demonstrate two facts more vividly than others. Firstly, the mechanism of improved transplant outcome by DST has not been elucidated, and, secondly, there is no good randomized study upon which to base the practice of DST. It is unlikely that the mechanism of action of DST is fully understood at present.

There are five major hypotheses which have been advanced to explain the beneficial effect of DST. The first and most straightforward is that donor-specific blood selects 'high responders' from amongst the potential recipients and this excludes them from transplantation. I have already considered this point briefly since most studies have produced strands of evidence against this hypothesis. To summarize the reasons for dismissing this hypothesis: patients who are excluded by humoral sensitization following DST include parous women and those who have been multiply transfused. These groups do not generally have poor transplant outcomes, and subsequent cadaver graft survival in those excluded from the living related transplant by DST is not worse than expected. Azathioprine reduces sensitization rates but does not affect survival rates which might be expected if it had reduced the ability of DST to select the responders. Finally, mixed lymphocyte culture (MLS) between donor and recipient following DST may demonstrate very strong responses in those who are transplanted successfully[71]. Selection is not a viable hypothesis.

A second hypothesis proposed was that DST leads to loss of specific anti-donor T cell clones, but it is possible to demonstrate the presence of anti-donor MLC responses in 77% of patients following DST[72]. Clonal deletion has its proponents, but it is hard to support it as the major mechanism for the effect of DST.

Non-cytotoxic antibodies which block Fc receptors can be demonstrated by an erythrocyte antibody rosette inhibition assay and have been shown to be associated with improved cadaveric transplantation after random blood transfusion[73]. Presence of these antibodies has also been demonstrated after DST in 9 of 25 patients tested, usually associated with previous pregnancy or transfusion with blood from third parties[74]. It is, however, uncertain whether the presence of these antibodies could explain the DST effect. Antibodies directed at T cell receptors specific for donor alloantigen, or to the idiotype of antibodies directed at donor HLA class I antigens (anti-idiotypic antibodies) have been demonstrated in serum taken from transplant recipients. Stimulation of these antibodies has been proposed as the mechanism for the blood transfusion effect[75] and for successful transplantation of patients with a peak positive crossmatch[76]. Investigation of this phenomenon in living related transplants has demonstrated the presence of anti-idiotypic antibodies in a minority of patients but has been unable to correlate their appearance after DST with good transplant outcome[77]. This hypothesis clearly awaits further evidence before it can reasonably be accepted or rejected.

Suppression of a variety of immune reponses in diverse situations can be attributed to suppressor cells[78]. It has been tempting to extend a hypothesis which invokes production of specific suppressor cells by DST to explain the beneficial effects seen after transplantation. Yielding to that temptation is the prerogative of hypothesis. Finding substantial support for the hypothesis is, however, still a task to be accomplished in clinical living related transplantation, though the indications appear to be favourable[79].

In conclusion, donor-specific transfusion for one haplotype and two haplotype mismatched living related transplantation and living unrelated transplantation, was the factor which was seen to improve survival rates sufficiently to justify the operations. Whether or not donor-specific transfusion is still required to achieve graft survival rates which exceed cadaveric transplant survival remains uncertain. There are proponents for both random third-party transfusion and no transfusion. Making a rational choice would be possible if either a recent randomized controlled trial were reported or the mechanisms of action were known. Until then, policies will have to be decided by less rational means, supported by selection of the literature.

LESSONS FROM EXPERIMENTAL MODELS

Animal models of transplantation have been fickle predictors of the outcome of clinical transplantation. This is true in the area of blood transfusion where the effect of blood transfusion in one model has not predicted the outcome of the same manœuvre in another model in the same species, let alone across species differences.

Donor antigens, in the form of blood transfusion, have been known to induce a state of unresponsiveness that is specific to those antigens. Tolerance of donor antigen can be acquired within 24 hours of birth in rodents, by injection of viable lymphopoietic cells. These animals can subsequently accept organ allografts bearing the histocompatibility antigens of the neonatally injected cells[80]. Donor-specific unresponsiveness to allografts can also be produced in some models by pretreatment with blood or various components of blood which express the incompatible histocompatibility antigens[81]. Many features of transfusion protocols have been explored in the rat. Fabre and Morris[82] used D Agouti (DA) and Lewis rat strains to demonstrate that multiple were more effective than single transfusions. Timing of the pretreatment was also significant with a seven-day interval between blood transfusion and transplantation producing optimum results. It was also demonstrated that choice of strains was crucial to outcome of the experiments. Lewis × DA F_1 transplants to Lewis yielded a more profound rejection response than the F_1 to DA. Choice of specificity control was equally important since pretreatment with DA blood in a Lewis recipient prolonged AS2 renal allograft survival, perhaps as a result of shared histocompatibility antigens between DA and AS2 strains. The degree to which these studies could not be extrapolated to the clinical situation was highlighted by the presence of donor-specific lymphocytotoxic antibodies, at the time of transplantation, without resultant hyperacute rejection. Transfusion of blood in dogs[83] and primates[84] has been shown to improve allograft survival but expense and lack of inbred strains has confined most experimental work to either the rat or, more recently, the mouse. Donor antigen has been given in many different forms with intravenous injection being more effective than intraperitoneal or subcutaneous routes. Purity of the transfused cell population has been the only, and, of necessity, imprecise, guide to the antigens relevant to modifying the host immune response. In a variety of different models, pure platelets[17], pure erythrocytes[85] and leukocytes[86] have all been both advocated and rejected; soluble antigen is, however, ineffective[87]. Rat erythrocytes express class I histocompatibility antigen but not class II. Purification of donor blood, such that a dose of 8×10^9 erythrocytes was contaminated with a mean of only 1.3 leukocytes, still yielded donor-specific suppression of renal allograft rejection[85]. Pure erythrocytes were only effective when given intravenously, did not alter survival of third-party allografts and had a dose-dependent effect. In the model used in that paper (Lewis to DA) class I antigens appeared to be sufficient to produce the 'transfusion effect' in the absence of class II. Human erythrocytes, in contrast to the rat, express very little class I antigen so one might not expect pure erythrocyte preparations to emulate the transfusion effect. A considerable proportion of the total class I antigen load in a unit of blood is, however, derived from the erythrocytes[88], thus swinging the argument back to proposing efficacy of pure red cell preparations for producing the transfusion effect. I have already discussed the actual findings in clinical practice.

Molecular genetic techniques have recently eludicated some of the possible reasons for the disparate results generated by previous studies. DNA-mediated transfer of genes coding for murine class I or class II histocompatibility antigens has allowed isolated foreign antigen to be expressed on L cells. A heterotopic mouse cardiac allograft model has been developed, with considerable technical skill and perseverance, to take advantage of well defined knowledge of the major histocompatibility complex in the mouse. It has thus been possible to merge these two developments to explore the role of injected isolated antigens for induction of immunological unresponsiveness to subsequent allografts[89]. In this study, individual genes coding for class I (H2-K or H2-D) and class II (H-2 IAα and H-2 IAβ) of C57 BL/10 mice were transfected into L cells from the C3H mouse. Varying doses of the transfected cells were injected intravenously into C3H mice and the effect on rejection of transplanted C57 BL/10 cardiac allografts measured. The data (Table 1.2) demonstrated unequivocal prolongation of allograft survival following pretreatment with a single donor-specific class I locus product, without the confusing effect of class II or minor histocompatibility antigens. Similarly, a class II product given one week before transplantation prolonged allograft survival significantly.

23

TABLE 1.2   Median survival time (MST) in days of C57 BL/10 (H-2^b) cardiac allografts in pretreated C3H (H-2^k) recipients

Pretreatment	MST (days)	Level of significance*
None	9.2	
Whole C57 BL/10 blood	34.2	
L cells untransfected	9.8	
L cells DWK-17†	8.8	
L cells I-A^k (C3H specific)	9.8	
L-D^b 10^7 cells	14.3	$p < 0.05$
L-K^b 10^7 cells	14.4	$p < 0.05$
5 × 10^6 cells	45.2	$p < 0.01$
2.5 × 10^6 cells	23.2	$p < 0.01$
L-IA^b 2.5 × 10^6 cells	14.7	$p < 0.05$
10^6 cells	19.6	$p < 0.01$

* Level of significance compared with no pretreatment.
† DWK-17 L cell clone transfected with an irrelevant chimaeric influenza haemagglutinin gene.
Data from Madsen et al. (1988). Nature (London), **332**, 161–164

The second feature of this model of the transfusion effect was that it enabled precise measurement of the quantity of antigen. Prolongation of graft survival was dose specific, such that both larger and smaller doses than those shown in Table 1.2 did not prolong survival. H-2K was more effective than either H2-D or H2-1A, at equivalent antigen loads, for modifying the immune response to subsequent transplantation. Perhaps most interesting was the fact that an optimum dose of H2-K was more effective even than whole blood in producing the 'transfusion effect'. The model suggests that the clinical observation of better graft survival after blood transfusion is due to sharing of HLA antigens between donors of blood and kidneys. This elegant experimental model of donor antigen pretreatment promises to unravel more of the mysteries surrounding the transfusion effect. The precision of cloned gene products is now the benchmark for future studies in this field but provides only the starting point of the investigation. The mechanism by which donor antigen actually modifies host immune responsiveness represents the next phase of study.

Transfusion of blood to rats has been shown not only to reduce the proliferative response, tested by MLC, of lymphocytes taken from thoracic duct drainage or lymph nodes, but to augment proliferation of splenic lymphocytes[90]. Donor-specific cytotoxicity measured by a ^{51}Cr-release assay was also markedly increased, suggesting that blood transfusion does not act by deletion of donor-specific cytotoxic clones. Furthermore, there is evidence that both azathioprine and cyclosporin, given at the time of blood transfusion, reduce the effect of the blood on subsequent rat cardiac allografts[91] and it thus seems certain that the mechanism must involve an active rather than passive phenomenon. Blood transfusion must abrogate cytotoxic effector cell function, either by induction of anti-idiotypic antibodies[92] or donor-specific suppressor cells[78]. The explanation seems likely to encompass both, rather than just one of these concepts.

MECHANISMS OF THE TRANSFUSION EFFECT IN CLINICAL PRACTICE

The selection theory

Selection of 'high responders' by blood transfusion has been proposed as a mechanism by which patients who produce antibodies in response to blood, are excluded from transplantation by a positive crossmatch test. These patients might, it is proposed, be the same group who respond to a kidney transplant by rejecting it. In discussion of the donor-specific transfusion effect, I have marshalled some arguments against this theory. It is similarly simplistic and incorrect with regard to the random transfusion effect. Significant sensitization is a rare phenomenon except in multiparous women, but the transfusion effect seen in clinical practice could not be explained by excluding that risk group[93,94]. The animal data that I have discussed in the previous section lent further support to antagonists of this theory.

Destruction of the theory of selection as the mechanism in clinical practice comes, in my view, from another quarter entirely. Blood transfusion has been associated with poor long-term outcome from surgery for colonic carcinoma which may be related to the surgical problems encountered when blood was required, or may be due to an effect of the blood transfusion on immune control of micrometastases[95]. Small aliquots of paternal blood have also been shown to influence the outcome of recurrent spontaneous abortion[96]. The effect of blood transfusion upon the immune system in these situations must be more profound than simply to induce antibodies which selectively halt transplantation. The final blow, if one is needed, is that the cytotoxic antibodies do not even select since they do not permanently prevent transplantation[46].

Fc receptor blocking antibodies

Antibodies which block membrane receptors for the Fc portion of IgG (Fc receptors) can be demonstrated in serum taken from patients before transplantation. These antibodies may be demonstrated by their capacity to inhibit rosette formation between the test B cells and ox or chicken erythrocytes coated with IgG. Erythrocyte rosette inhibition has been shown to be a function of non-cytotoxic IgG antibodies and resides in the $F(ab')_2$ and not Fc portion[73]. Other studies have suggested that a blocking factor may also be present in a high molecular weight fraction of serum[97]. Development of receptor-blocking antibody has been demonstrated following blood transfusion[98] and correlates with transplant survival in some[73] but not all studies[97]. A prospective study of matching donors and recipients for erythrocyte rosette inhibition activity has demonstrated a possible beneficial effect in recipients of first cadaver grafts, particularly when poorly matched at HLA-DR[99]. It is, therefore, possible that some of the effect of transfusion may relate to stimulation of these non-cytotoxic antibodies.

Suppressor lymphocytes

Most of the evidence supporting the role of suppressor T lymphocytes has accrued from experimental models of transfusion and transplantation[78]. Much of this evidence is persuasive and seductive in its elegance, such that it is hard to deny to T lymphocytes a role that suppresses and regulates the activity of T helper cells. Suppressor cells can be taken from the spleen of a rat bearing a successfully transplanted allogeneic kidney (survival having been achieved by trans-

26

fusion or immunosuppression) and then given to a fresh recipient which will specifically accept an identical allogeneic kidney as given to the first animal. This demonstration is hampered by the fact that it is necessary to irradiate lightly the second host to be able to see the results of the cell transfer. Clinical evidence, by contrast, is sparse and inelegant.

A recipient of a cadaveric transplant mismatched at two HLA-A, one-B and two-DR antigens was studied in detail when, despite withdrawal of immunosuppression because of hepatitis, sustained tolerance of the graft was apparent[100]. The mixed lymphocyte response of T cells taken from the recipient before the transplant and donor lymphocytes could be suppressed by the addition of recipient cells taken after the transplant. The suppressive activity was shown to be donor specific when nylon wool-adherent T lymphocytes were added but non-specific when non-adherent cells were added. Mixed lymphocyte responses could also be suppressed by serum taken from the recipient after transplantation. This suppressive factor was shown to be IgG, specific for the HLA type of the recipient, and effective when added to the responder and not the stimulator donor cells. Other investigators have characterized cells which may act as mediators of specific unresponsiveness in patients with successful renal allografts[101], but there has been no substantive evidence that these phenomena arise from blood transfusions.

Anti-idiotypic antibodies

It has been postulated that the beneficial effect of transfusion may be mediated by a 'two stage process' in which it is envisaged that suppressor cells are induced initially and that anti-idiotype antibodies provide suppression in the second stages[102].

The unique structure of each immunoglobulin variable region which determines the specificity of an antibody, the idiotype, may itself be recognized by a second anti-idiotypic antibody which may then regulate the effects of the first antibody. These anti-idiotypic antibodies have been identified after blood transfusions in patients awaiting renal transplantation[103], confirming the results of animal experiments[92]. That they may have some role in modifying the response to an allograft in the clinical situation is a suggestion that has only recently been given backing. Reed and her colleagues have shown that anti-idiotypic antibodies may be a factor in the successful transplantation of patients with a peak-serum positive crossmatch[76]. In their study, nine of ten patients, with a positive crossmatch using historical peak-serum samples and a successful transplant, had antibodies (anti-idiotypic antibodies) present in serum taken at the time of transplantation, which inhibited the positive crossmatch. By contrast, nine of ten patients whose grafts failed after a peak positive crossmatch transplant had antibodies which potentiated the cytotoxic effect of the peak-serum sample. There is thus some evidence linking antibodies which suppress mixed lymphocyte responses or inhibit cytotoxic antibodies and blood transfusion. Separate strands link those antibodies to tolerance of a graft, albeit in a rather special situation. It is clearly possible that the blood transfusion effect may, to some extent and in some patients, be explained by stimulation of anti-idiotypic antibodies.

A BLOOD TRANSFUSION POLICY

No transfusion policy can satisfy its critics since, as I have tried to demonstrate, there are sufficiently conflicting reports to ensure debate on every issue. Description of a blood transfusion policy is appended here as little more than an illustration of the factors which need decision. By the date of publication, this policy may have been altered by experience, new data, or by rereading of old data, but the questions requiring decision will probably not have changed.

Elective transfusion of untransfused potential transplant recipients

It is, in my view, premature to discard the sturdy prop which supported transplant survival rates in the late 1970s and early 1980s. Untransfused recipients should, therefore, be transfused. The exception to this rule is the parous women who will be at significant risk of developing high levels of humoral sensitization. It is possible to turn the argument around and take comfort in data which suggest the penalty for not transfusing these patients will, at worst, be small.

Packed cells, between three and ten days after donation are a standard blood preparation which has the virtues of simplicity, availability and demonstrated efficacy. Three units are certainly sufficient to gain most, if not all, of the benefit derived from transfusion at about three-fifths of the risk of five units. Intervals of two weeks between tranfusions have the hallmark of historical precedent and organizational simplicity. Patients may thus be placed on the active transplant waiting list within ten weeks, if one allows four weeks after the last transfusion to detect development of cytotoxic antibodies. Men and nulliparous women are at low risk of developing high levels of panel reactivity with three transfusions, and the clumsy procedure of screening antibodies between each unit of blood can therefore be dispensed with.

Elective transfusion of previously transfused patients

The risk of sensitization by blood transfusion in patients who have been given blood at some time in the past is higher than for the untransfused. In contrast, therefore, neurotic attention to panel reactive antibody levels is probably warranted, and use of flow cytometry techniques a justifiable luxury, given access.

Patients previously transfused with only one unit of blood, or those in whom the transfusion history is incomplete, should receive blood electively, unless they are parous or already have lymphocytotoxic antibodies. In the latter situation, I still transfuse two or three units if the panel reactivity is low (less than 20%) but measure antibodies two weeks after each unit and stop if the level rises above 20%.

Some patients have been given multiple transfusions many years before they present for renal transplantation. Parity is again an absolute contraindication to further elective transfusions, as are high levels of panel reactive antibodies, because of the risk of sensitization. There is evidence to support the efficacy of blood transfused two years before a transplant, but insufficient data to examine more distant time periods. An arbitrary time interval separates multiply transfused patients considered (greater than ten years between transplantation and previous transfusions) and patients not considered (less than ten years) for further elective transfusions. Panel reactive antibodies cytotoxic to more than 20% of the panel provides a further arbitrary division, as above, between those given up to three elective transfusions and those not.

Living related transplant recipients

Parous women, patients previously given multiple third party transfusions, and recipients who have lost a previous transplant, will be likely to be sensitized by donor-specific blood whether given azathioprine or not. These patients are therefore not given either random or donor-specific blood before the living related graft. Untransfused recipients will probably benefit from a unit of donor blood divided into three aliquots and given at two week intervals. Azathioprine at a dose of $2.0 \, \text{mg} \, \text{kg}^{-1} \, \text{d}^{-1}$ may be started one week before the first transfusion and continue until the transplant, at which time I currently use triple therapy with cyclosporin, prednisolone and azathioprine at reduced dose. I would not transplant across a positive crossmatch due to antibodies against either donor HLA class I or class II antigens.

Clinical requirement for transfusion

Clinical indications for blood transfusion will continue to occur despite the increasing availability of erythropoietin. Evidence is progressively accumulating which suggests that repetitive transfusion of the 'transfusion-dependent anephric patient' is the factor which often causes persistence of the highly sensitized state. Erythropoietin can be expected to solve this problem, but it will be interesting to discover how well these patients fare with current-serum negative, peak-serum positive crossmatch transplants. For the majority of individuals with a single urgent indication for transfusion, the risks to the patient of withholding blood have to be balanced against the risks of sensitization. A fourth unit of blood in a patient who was not sensitized by the previous three units provides a very small risk of rendering them untransplantable. A unit of blood given to a moderately sensitized multiparous patient, or to someone who has rejected their first graft and developed antibodies, is likely to yield a considerable adverse

30

effect upon their chances of subsequent transplantation. Cotton wool leukocyte filtration of blood may reduce the bulk of transfused antigen sufficiently to reduce sensitization rates without incurring a clinical penalty, though it does of course add to the cost.

Transfusion of blood at the time of, or soon after, graft rejection is probably the most efficient way of rendering a patient persistently highly sensitized. In young patients, therefore, anaemia should be symptomatic before a blood transfusion is given.

FUTURE PROSPECTS

Randomized controlled trials and continued international registration of results promise to provide a more secure basis upon which some decisions may be made. Application of molecular genetic techniques has begun to yield fine dissection of both animal models of the transfusion effect and polymorphisms of HLA. Advances in both these fields can certainly be expected to spill over into the complexities of clinical decision making. The effects of HLA class II matched and mismatched transfusions are, for example, under investigation and may prove of interest. It would be an unwise person who predicted the transfusion policies of five or ten years hence, except to comment that the five- and ten-year results of current practices will probably influence those policies. The issue of blood transfusion in clinical transplantation is unlikely to be consigned to medical history.

REFERENCES

1. Kissmeyer-Nielsen, F., Olsen, S., Petersen, V.P. and Fjeldborg, O. (1966). Hyperacute rejection of kidney allografts associated with pre-existing humoral antibodies against donor cells. *Lancet*, 1, 662–665
2. Dausset, J. (1955). Leuco-agglutinins. IV. Leucoagglutinins and blood transfusions. *Vox Sang*, 4, 190–198
3. Patel, R. and Terasaki, P.I. (1969). Significance of the positive crossmatch test in kidney transplantation. *N. Engl. J. Med.*, 280, 735–739
4. Michielsen, P. (1966). Hemodialyse at transplantation renale. *Proc. Eur. Dial. Transplant. Assoc.*, 3, 162–164
5. Dossetor, J.B., MacKinnon, K.J., Gault, M.H. and MacLean, L.D. (1967). Cadaver kidney transplants. *Transplantation,* 5, 844–853.

6. Morris, P. J., Ting, A. and Stocker, J. (1968). Leukocyte antigens in renal transplantation. I The paradox of blood transfusions in renal transplantation. *Med. J. Aust*, **2**, 1088–1090
7. Hume, D. I., Rapaport, F. T. and Dausset, J. (eds). *Kidney Transplantation*, p. 131. (New York: Grune and Stratton)
8. Opelz, G., Sengar, D. P. S., Mickey, M. R. and Terasaki, P. I. (1973). Effect of blood transfusions on subsequent kidney transplants. *Transplant. Proc.*, **5**, 253–259
9. Opelz, G. For the Collaborative transplant study (1987). Improved kidney graft survival in non-transfused recipients. *Transplant. Proc.*, **19**, 149–152
10. Van Rood, J. J. (1983). Pretransplant blood transfusion: sure! but how and why? (1983). *Transplant. Proc.*, **15**, 915–916
11. Opelz, G. (1984). Blood transfusion. In Morris, P. J. (ed.) *Kidney Transplantation, Principles and Practice*, Edn 2, pp. 323–334. (New York: Grune and Stratton)
12. Opelz, G. (1988). To transfuse or not before transplantation. In Morris, P. J. (ed.) *Kidney Transplantation, Principles and Practice*, Edn 3. (New York: Grune and Stratton)
13. Opelz, G. and Terasaki, P. I. (1978). Improvement of kidney-graft survival with increased numbers of blood transfusion. *N. Engl. J. Med.*, **299**, 799–803
14. Cecka, M. and Cicciarelli, J. (1985). The transfusion effect. In Terasaki, P. I. (ed.) *Clinical Kidney Transplants*, pp. 73–92 (UCLA: Tissue Typing Laboratory)
15. Persijn, G. G., Van Leeuwen, A., Parlevliet, J., Cohen, B., Lansbergen Q., D'Amaro, J. and Van Rood, J. J. (1981). Two major factors influencing kidney graft survival in Eurotransplant: HLA-DR matching and blood transfusions. *Transplant. Proc.*, **13**, 150–154
16. Fuller, T. C., Delmonico, F. L., Cosini, A. B., Huggins, G. E., King, M. and Russell, P. S. (1978). Impact of blood transfusion on renal transplantation. *Ann. Surg.*, **187**, 211–218
17. Batchelor, J. R., Welsh, K. I. and Burgos, H. (1977). Immunological enhancement. *Transplant. Proc.*, **9**, 931–936
18. Borleffs, J. C. C., Neuhaus, P., Van Rood, J. J. and Balner, H. (1982). Platelet transfusions improve kidney allograft survival in rhesus monkeys without inducing cytotoxic antibodies. *Lancet*, **1**, 1117–1118
19. Oh, J. H., McClure, H. M. and Tuttle, E. P. (1983). Immunological unresponsiveness induced by platelet transfusion in rhesus monkeys. *Transplantation*, **36**, 727–728
20. Errett, L. E., Allen, N., Deierhoi, M. H., Denton, T. G., Wood, R. F. M. and Morris, P. J. (1985). The effect of platelet transfusions on renal allograft survival and sensitisation in dogs. *Tissue Antigens*, **25**, 28–32
21. Marquet, R. L., Tank, B., Jeineman, E., Obertop, H., Niessen, G. J. C. M., Bignen, A. B., Westbroek, D. L. and Jeekel, J. (1983). Pre-transplant platelet transfusions do not improve kidney graft survival in beagle dogs. *Lancet*, **1**, 774
22. Chapman, J. R., Ting, A., Fisher, M., Carter, N. P. and Morris, P. J. (1986). Failure of platelet transfusion to improve human renal allograft survival. *Transplantation*, **41**, 468–473
23. Pallardo, L. N., Montoro, J., Moll, J. L., Sanchez, J., Soler, M. A., Marty, M. and Cruz, J. N. (1985). Platelet transfusions do not improve cadaveric renal allograft survival. *Transplant. Proc.*, **17**, 2338–2339

24. Betuel, H., Cantarovitch, D., Robert, F., Gebuher, L., Touraine, J. L., Dubernard, J. N. and Traeger, J. (1985). Platelet transfusions preparative for kidney transplantation. *Transplant. Proc.*, **17**, 2335–2337

25. Norman, D. J., Barry, J. N., Durr, M. and Wetesteon, P. (1985). A preliminary analysis of a randomised study of buffy coat transfusions in renal transplantation. *Transplant. Proc.*, **17**, 2330–2332

26. Okazaki, H., Takahashi, H., Miura, K., Makoto, I. and Taguchi, Y. (1984). Significant reduction of sensitisation and improved allograft outcome with donor specific buffy coat transfusions. *Transplantation*, **37**, 523–525

27. Ferrara, G. B., Tosi, R. N., Azzolina, G., Carminati, G. and Longo, A. (1974). HL-A unresponsiveness induced by weekly transfusions of small aliquots of whole blood. *Transplantation*, **17**, 194–200

28. Muller, J. Y., Kaplan, C., Betuel, H., Bignon, J. D., Fauchet, R., Gluckman, J. C., Soulillou, J. P. and Thibault, Ph. (1982). Effet des transfusions sanguines sur les graffes de vein. *Nouv. Presse Med.*, **11**, 3697–3701

29. Stiller, C. R., Lockwood, B. L. and Sinclair, N. R. (1978). Beneficial effect of operation-day blood-transfusions on human allograft survival. *Lancet*, **1**, 169–170

30. Williams, K. A., Ting, A., French, M. E., Oliver, D. and Morris, P. J. (1980). Peroperative blood-transfusions improve cadaveric renal-allograft survival in non-transfused recipients. *Lancet*, **1**, 1104–1106

31. Sanfilippo, F., Spees, E. K. and Vaughn, W. K. (1984). The timing of pretransplant transfusions and renal allograft survival. *Transplantation*, **37**, 344–350

32. Heineman, E., Marquet, R. L., Heystek, G. A., Cobussen, A. and Jeekel, J. (1983). Modification of allograft rejection in rates by blood transfusions to the donor. *Transplant. Proc.*, **15**, 994–996

33. Jeekel, J., Harder, F., Persijn, G. G., Brynger, H. and Marquet, R. L. (1983). Beneficial effect of blood transfusion to the donor on kidney graft survival in man: a study in three centers. *Transplant. Proc.*, **15**, 973–975

34. Frisk, B., Berglin, E. and Brynger, H. (1983). Transfused cadaver kidney donors and graft survival. *Transplantation*, **35**, 352

35. Cecka, M. and Terasaki, P. I. (1987). Improvement of kidney transplant regraft results by using trauma death donors. *Transplantation*, **44**, 792–795

36. Voronoy, Y. Y. (1936). Sobre el bloque del aparato reticloendothelial del hombre en alaqunas formes de intoxicacion por el sublimado y sobre la transplantation del rinon cadaverico como metodo de tratamiento de la anuria consecutiva a aquella intoxicacion. *Siglo. Med.*, **97**, 296

37. Rubin, R. H., Jenkins, R. L., Shaw, B. W., Shaffer, D., Pearl, R. H., Erb, S., Nonaco, A. P. and van Thiel, D. H. (1987). The acquired immunodeficiency syndrome and transplantation. *Transplantation*, **44**, 1–4

38. Melzer, J. S., Husing, R. M., Feduska, N. J., Tomlanovich, S. J., Vincenti, F., Amend, W. J. C., Garovoy, M. and Salvatierra, O. (1987). The beneficial effect of pretransplant blood transfusions in cyclosporine-treated cadaver renal allograft recipients. *Transplantation*, **43**, 61–64

39. Dausset, J., Nenna, A. and Brecy, A. (1954). Leukoagglutinins, V. *Blood*, **9**, 696–720

40. Opelz, G., Mickey, M. R. and Terasaki, P. I. (1981). Blood transfusions and kidney transplants: remaining controversies. *Transplant. Proc.*, **13**, 136–141

33

41. Opelz, G., Graver, B., Mickey, R. and Terasaki, P. I. (1981). Lymphocytotoxic antibody responses to transfusions in potential kidney transplant recipients. *Transplantation*, **32**, 177–183
42. Scornik, J. C., Ireland, J. E., Howard, R. J. and Pfaff, W. W. (1987). Assessment of the risk for broad sensitization by blood transfusions. *Transplantation*, **37**, 249–253
43. Scornik, J. C., Ireland, J. E., Salomon, D. R., Howard, R. J., Fennell, R. S. and Pfaff, W. W. (1987). Pretransplant blood transfusions in patients with previous pregnancies. *Transplantation*, **43**, 449–450
44. Sanfilippo, F., Vaughn, W. K., Bollinger, R. R. and Spees, E. K. (1984). The influence of pretransplant transfusions, using different blood products, on patient sensitization and renal allograft survival. *Transplantation*, **37**, 350–356
45. Rafftery, M. J., Lang, C. J., Schwarz, G., O'Shea, J., Varghese, Z., Sweny, P., Fernando, O. N. and Moorhead, J. F. (1985). Failure of azathropine to prevent sensitization due to third-party transfusion. *Transplant. Proc.*, **17**, 1044–1046
46. Cardella, C. J., Falk, J. A., Peters, P., Nicholson, J. and Harding, N. (1982). Do repeated blood transfusions prevent successful transplantation in highly sensitized potential transplant recipients? *Transplant. Proc.*, **14**, 359–60
47. Norman, D. J., Barry, J. M., Boehne, C. and Wetzsteon, P. (1985). Natural history of patients who make cytotoxic antibodies following prospective fresh blood transfusions. *Transplant. Proc.*, **17**, 1041–1043
48. Sanfilippo, F., Vaughn, W. K., Bollinger, R. R. and Spees, E. K. (1982). Comparative effects of pregnancy, transfusion, and prior graft rejection on sensitization and renal transplant results. *Transplantation*, **34**, 360–366
49. Chapman, J. R., Taylor, C. J., Ting, A. and Morris, P. J. (1986). Immunoglobulin class and specificity of antibodies causing positive T cell crossmatches. *Transplantation*, **42**, 608–613
50. Sanfilippo, F., Goeken, N., Niblack, G., Scornik, J. and Vaughn, W. K. (1987). The effect of first cadaver renal transplant HLA–A,B match on sensitization levels and retransplant rates following graft failure. *Transplantation*, **43**, 240–244
51. Chapman, J. R. (1986). Humoral sensitisation of potential renal transplant recipients. *M.D. Thesis.* Cambridge University
52. Scornik, J. C., Ireland, J. E., Howard, R. J., Pfaff, W. W. and Fennell, R. S. (1983). Sensitization by blood transfusion in previously transplanted patients. *Transplantation*, **35**, 505–506
53. Lundgren, G., Groth, C. G., Albrechtsen, D., Brynger, H., Flatmark, A., Frodin, L., Gabel, H., Husberg, B., Klintmalm, G., Maurer, W., Persson, H., and Thorsby, E. (1986). HLA-matching and pretransplant blood transfusions in cadaveric renal transplantation – a changing picture with cyclosporin. *Lancet*, **2**, 66–69
54. Opelz, G. (1987). Improved kidney graft survival in nontransfused recipients. *Transplant. Proc.*, **19**, 149–152
55. Groth, C. G. (1987). There is no need to give blood transfusions as pretreatment for renal transplantation in the cyclosporine era. *Transplant. Proc.*, **19**, 153–154
56. Terasaki, P. I., Himaya, N. S., Cecka, M., Cicciarelli, J., Cook, D. J., Ito, T., Iwaki, Y., Mickey, R., Takiff, H., Tiwari, J. L. and Toyotome, A. (1986). In Terasaki, P. I. (ed.) *Clinical Transplants 1986*, pp. 367–92. (Los Angeles: UCLA Tissue Typing Laboratory)

57. Newton, W. T. and Anderson, C. B. (1973). Planned pre-immunization of renal allograft recipients. *Surgery*, **74**, 430
58. Salvatierra, O., Vincenti, F., Amend, W., Potter, D., Iwaki, Y., Opelz, G., Terasaki, P., Duca, R., Cochrum, K., Hanes, D., Stoney, R. J. and Feduska, N. J. (1980). Deliberate donor specific blood transfusions prior to living related renal transplantation. *Ann. Surg.*, **192**, 543–552
59. Glass, N. R., Miller, D. T., Sollinger, H. W. and Belzer, F. O. (1983). Comparative analysis of the DST and Imuran-plus-DST protocols for live donor renal transplantation. *Transplantation*, **36**, 636–641
60. Colombe, B. W., Lou, D. D., Salvatierra, O. and Garavoy, M. R. (1987). Two patterns of sensitization demonstrated by recipients of donor-specific transfusion. *Transplantation*, **44**, 509–515
61. Vaidya, S., Sommer, B. G., Pagel, E., Koegel, M. and Ferguson, R. M. (1986). Assessment of factors associated with donor-specific sensitization in patients given donor-specific blood transfusions. *Transplantation*, **42**, 695–697
62. Salvatierra, O., Melzer, J., Potter, D., Garavoy, M., Vincenti, F., Amend, W. J. C., Husing, R., Hopper, S. and Feduska, N. J. (1985). A seven-year experience with donor-specific blood transfusions. *Transplantation*, **40**, 654–659
63. Okazaki, H., Takahashi, H., Oguma, S., Jimbo, M. and Ishizaki, M. (1987). Transplant outcome of desensitised recipients after donor specific transfusion. *Transplant. Proc.*, **19**, 750–752
64. Whelchel, J. D., Shaw, J. F., Curtis, J. J., Luke, R. G. and Diethelm, A. G. (1982). Effect of pretransplant stored donor-specific blood transfusions on early renal allograft survival in one-haplotype living related transplants. *Transplantation*, **34**, 326–329
65. Cheigh, J. S., Suthanthiran, M., Kaplan, M., Evelyn, M., Riggio, R. R., Fotino, M., Schechter, N., Wolf, C. F. W., Stubenbord, W. T., Stenzel, K. H. and Rubin, A. L. (1984). Induction of immune alterations and successful renal transplantation with a simplified method of donor-specific blood transfusion. *Transplantation*, **38**, 501–506
66. Schweizer, R. T., Bartus, S. A., Rorelli, M. A. and Bow, L. M. (1986). Use of two donor-specific transfusions for living-related donor kidney transplantation. *Transplantation*, **42**, 562–564
67. Flechner, S. N., Kerman, R. H., Van Buren, C. and Kahan, B. D. (1984). Successful transplantation of cyclosporin-treated haploidentical living-related renal recipients without blood transfusions. *Transplantation*, **37**, 73–76
68. Albrechtsen, D., Flatmark, A., Lundgren, G., Brynger, H., Frodin, L., Groth, C. G., Gabel, H. and Thorsby, E. (1987). Renal transplantation from HLA-haploidentical living related donors: The Scandinavian multicenter study of the effects of cyclosporin immunosuppression. *Clin. Transplant.*, **1**, 104–107
69. Opelz, G. (1985). Comparison of random transfusions with donor-specific transfusions for pretreatment of HLA One-haplotype-matched related donor kidney transplant recipients. *Transplant. Proc.*, **17**, 2357–2361
70. Iwaki, Y. and Terasaki, P. I. (1986). Donor specific transfusion. In Terasaki, P. I. (ed.) *Clinical Transplants 1986*, pp. 267–275. (Los Angeles: UCLA Tissue Typing Laboratory)
71. Burlingham, W. J., Grailer, A., Sparks-Mackety, E. N. F., Sondel, P. M. and Sollinger, H. W. (1987). Improved renal allograft survival following donor-specific transfusions. *Transplantation*, **43**, 41–46

72. Bakran, A., Taylor, G. M., Read, I., Fergusson, W. and Johnson, R. W. G. (1987). Donor-specific T cell alloreactivity in relation to 1 haplotype-mismatched blood transfusion prior to living-donor renal transplantation. *Transplant. Proc.*, **19**, 748–749

73. MacLeod, A. M., Mason, R. J., Stewart, K. N., Power, D. A., Shewan, W. G., Edward, N. and Catto, G. R. D. (1982). Association of Fc receptor-blocking antibodies and human renal transplant survival. *Transplantation*, **34**, 273–279

74. MacLeod, A. M., Hillis, A. N., Mather, A., Bone, J. N. and Catto, G. R. D. (1987). Effect of cyclosporin, previous third-party transfusion, and pregnancy on antibody development after donor-specific transfusion before renal transplantation. *Lancet*, **1**, 416–418

75. Singal, D. P., Fagnilli, L. and Joseph, S. (1983). Blood transfusions induce anti-idiotypic antibodies in renal transplant patients. *Transplant. Proc.*, **15**, 1005–1008

76. Reed, E., Hardy, M., Benvenisty, A., Lattes, C., Brensilver, J., McCabe, R., Reemsta, K., King, D. W. and Suciu-Foca, N. (1987). Effect of anti-idiotypic antibodies to HLA on graft survival in renal allograft recipients. *N. Engl. J. Med.*, **316**, 1450–1455

77. Toma, H., Hayasaka, Y., Yasuo, N., Takahashi, K., Teraoka; S. and Ota, K. (1987). Anti-idiotypic autoantibodies after donor-specific blood transfusions. *Transplant. Proc.*, **19**, 755–757

78. Hutchinson, I. V. (1986). Suppressor T cells in allogeneic models. *Transplantation*, **41**, 547–555

79. Leivestad, T. and Thorsby, E. (1984). Effects of HLA-haploidentical blood transfusions on donor-specific immune responsiveness. *Transplantation*, **37**, 175–181

80. Billingham, R. E., Brent, L. and Medawar, P. B. (1953). Actively acquired tolerance of foreign cells. *Nature (London)*, **172**, 603–606

81. Medawar, P. B. (1963). The use of antigenic tissue extracts to weaken the immunological reaction against skin homografts in mice. *Transplantation*, **1**, 21–57

82. Fabre, J. W. and Morris, P. J. (1972). The effect of donor strain blood pre-treatment on renal allograft rejection in rats. *Transplantation*, **14**, 608–617

83. Van der Linden, C. J., Burman, W. A., Vegt, P. A., Greep, J. M. and Jeekel, J. (1982). Effect of blood transfusions on canine renal allograft survival. *Transplantation*, **33**, 400–402

84. Van Es, A. A., Marquet, R. L., Van Rood, J. J. and Balmer, H. (1978). Influence of a single blood transfusion in unrelated rhesus monkeys. *Transplantation*, **26**, 325–330

85. Wood, K. J., Evins, J. and Morris, P. J. (1985). Suppression of renal allograft rejection in the rat by class I antigens on purified erythrocytes. *Transplantation*, **39**, 56–62

86. Lauchart, W., Alkins, B. J. and Davies, D. A. L. (1980). Only B lymphocytes induce active enhancement of rat cardiac allografts. *Transplantation*, **29**, 259–261

87. Spencer, S. C. and Fabre, J. (1987). Bulk purification of a naturally occurring soluble form of RT1-A class I major histocompatibility complex antigen from DA rat liver, and studies of specific immunosuppression. *Transplantation*, **44**, 141–148

88. Everett, S. T., Kao, K-J. and Scornik, J. C. (1987). Class I HLA molecules on human erythrocytes. *Transplantation*, **44**, 123–129
89. Madsen, J. C., Superina, R. A., Wood, K. J. and Morris, P. J. (1988). Immunological unresponsiveness induced by recipient cells transfected with donor MHC genes. *Nature (London)*, **332**, 161–164
90. Quigley, R. L., Wood, K. J. and Morris, P. J. (1988). Investigation of the mechanism of active enhancement of renal allograft survival by blood transfusion. *Immunology*, **63**, 373–381
91. Johnson, C. P., Munda, R., Alexander, J. W., Balakrishnan, K. and Blanton, M. (1984). The effect of donor-specific transfusions on rat heart allograft survival. *Transplantation*, **38**, 575–578
92. Ludwin, D., Joseph, S. and Singal, D. P. (1986). MLC-Inhibiting antibodies in mice after blood transfusions. *Transplantation*, **41**, 100–104
93. Opelz, G., Graver, B. and Terasaki, P. I. (1981). Induction of high kidney graft survival rate by multiple transfusion. *Lancet*, **1**, 1223–1225
94. Feduska, N. J., Vincenti, F., Amend, W. J., Duca, R., Cochrum, K. and Salvatierra, O. (1979). Do blood transfusions enhance the possibility of a compatible transplant? *Transplantation*, **27**, 35–38
95. Blumberg, N., Heal, J. M., Murphy, P., Agarwal, M. M. and Chuang, C. (1986). Association between transfusion of whole blood and recurrence of cancer. *Br. Med. J.*, **293**, 530–533
96. Mowbray, J. F., Gibbings, C. R., Sidgwick, A. S., Ruszkiewicz, M. and Beard, R. W. (1983). Effects of transfusion in women with recurrent spontaneous abortion. *Transplant. Proc.*, **15**, 896–899
97. Forwell, M. A., Cocker, J. E., Peel, M. G., Tsakiris, D. J., Briggs, J. D., Junor, B. J. R., MacSween, R. N. M. and Sandilands, G. P. (1987). Correlation between high-molecular-weight Fcγ-receptor-blocking factors in serum and renal allograft survival. *Transplantation*, **44**, 227–233
98. Macleod, A. M., Power, D. A., Mason, R. J., Stewart, K. N., Shewan, W. G., Edward, N. and Catto, G. R. (1982). Possible mechanism of action of transfusion effect in renal transplantation. *Lancet*, **2**, 468–470
99. Macleod, A. M., Stewart, K. N., Mather, A., Engeset, J., Edward, N. and Catto, G. R. D. (1987). Noncytotoxic antibodies and renal transplant outcome. *Transplantation*, **44**, 840–842
100. Suzuki, S., Mizuochi, I., Sada, M. and Ameoniya, H. (1985). Transplantation tolerance mediated by suppressor T cells and suppressive antibody in a recipient of a renal transplant. *Transplantation*, **40**, 357–363
101. Charpentier, B. M., Bach, M. A., Lang, P. and Fries, D. (1983). Expression of OKT8 antigen and Fcr receptors by suppressor cells mediating specific unresponsiveness between recipient and donor in renal-allograft-tolerant patients. *Transplantation*, **36**, 495–501
102. Woodruff, M. F. A. and van Rood, J. J. (1983). Possible implications of the effect of blood transfusion on allograft survival. *Lancet*, **1**, 1201–1203
103. Barkley, S. C., Sakai, R. S., Ettenger, R. B., Fine, R. N. and Jordan, S. C. (1987). Determination of anti-idiotypic antibodies to anti-HLA IgG following blood transfusions. *Transplantation*, **44**, 30–34

37

88. Thwait S.T., Sass G.L. and Bergmann L.W. (1987) Oligo-RNA selectivity on adenine deaminase. *Transplantation*, 43, 321-329.

89. Vaughan P.J., Suppiah S.A., Wood K.J. and Morris P.J. (1988) Immun-...

90. Opelz G.L., Wood K.J. and Morris P.J. (1988) Immunization of the recipient...

91. Gibson C.D., Morris P.J., Shepards G.W., Bankgardner R. and Simpson A. (1988)...

92. Hutchinson I.V., Tilney D.J. and Sironi P.J. (1990)...

93. Cook G.D. Garvey D. and Yamada P.J. (1988)...

94. Feldman S.J., Koopman D., Oksman W.A., Dixon K., Cochran R. and van...

95. Ishikawa M., Hara J., Matsui P., Aozuka M.M. and Crump C.J. (1988)...

96. Morris T., Mabbott L., Brown S.R., Ridgemore K. and Bland R.W. (1987)...

97. Farwell M.A., Parker E.B., Paul M.C., Tobin D.D., Gray I.D., Parker H.T., McEwen K.S.M. and Santamala C.D. (1987)...

98. Monaco A.W., Hoopes T.A., Mason L.D., Brown S.K., Buckwater W.C., Tucker M.N. and Chang C.F. (1985)...

99. Hancks M.H., Hewett M.B., Kumar K.K. Hoopes J.T., Orion C.C. and...

100. Smith S.J., Winterburn S.S.R. and Anderson J.D. (1989)...

101. Gunter J.B.M., Glass M., Lamb P. and Roop K.S. (1987)...

102. Glover M.J., Hutchison D.J. (1987)...

103. Francis S.J., Fagg R.S., Morton R.B., Bradley K.B. and Jenner M. (1987)...

2
THE HIGHLY SENSITIZED PATIENT

A. TING

Patients waiting for kidney transplantation may become sensitized to histocompatibility (HLA) antigens as a result of pregnancies, blood transfusions or a previous failed graft. This sensitization is evidenced by the presence of HLA antibodies in the sera of these patients. Conventionally, patients waiting for renal transplantation are screened for the presence of these antibodies on a regular basis by testing their sera against lymphocytes in a cytotoxic test. The lymphocyte target panels are usually unseparated lymphocytes from the peripheral blood (PBL) of normal individuals, but may also include separated T and B lymphocytes from the PBL of normal volunteers, and B lymphocytes from chronic lymphatic leukaemia patients (CLL cells).

In the mid-1960s, a number of laboratories found, in retrospective studies, that a kidney transplant performed in a patient who had cytotoxic antibodies in pregraft sera which reacted with the lymphocytes of the donor was likely to be hyperacutely rejected[1,2]. On the basis of these observations, the performance of a crossmatch test prior to transplantation was deemed mandatory, and a positive crossmatch was considered a strict contraindication to transplantation (the crossmatch dogma). The adoption of this dogma has meant that patients who develop broadly reactive antibodies (highly sensitized patients) are difficult to transplant because they will give a positive crossmatch with most potential kidney donors. These patients have to wait a very long time for an appropriate donor or are not transplanted at all and have to remain on long-term dialysis.

The criteria for the definition of a highly sensitized patient vary from one laboratory to another. Some laboratories consider patients with antibodies reacting with the lymphocytes of as little as 50% of a random panel as being highly sensitized[3]. On the other hand, our laboratory considers patients with antibodies which react with at least 90% of the target panel members as being highly sensitized. We feel that this 'strict' definition is more appropriate because it selects out those patients who are difficult to transplant if standard crossmatch procedures are used. It is this ˜roup of patients for whom special protocols need to be implemented if they are to be successfully transplanted.

Before discussing the methods which have been implemented to try to transplant these patients, I shall briefly discuss two topics which are central to the problems of the highly sensitized patient, and these are: the causes of high sensitization and how this can be prevented.

CAUSES OF HIGH SENSITIZATION

Although pregnancies and blood transfusions can cause sensitization to HLA antigens, it is rare for each alone to cause patients to become highly sensitized. The causes of high sensitization are blood transfusions in women who have had previous pregnancies, multiple blood transfusions alone, or a previous failed graft[4]; it is well recognized that it is the latter which is the main cause of highly sensitized patients.

Some patients develop broadly reactive lymphocytotoxic antibodies without any apparent overt antigenic challenge, and it has been speculated that viral infections may be a cause[5,6]. These antibodies usually react with the patient's own lymphocytes and their specificity is not directed at HLA antigens. In addition, they can react with 80–100% of a random panel and these patients are then categorized as highly sensitized.

PREVENTION OF HIGH SENSITIZATION

To achieve this objective, the three causes of sensitization would have to be reduced or prevented; namely, pregnancies, blood transfusions and graft failure. Prevention of pregnancies, obviously, is not something to consider, although a sensible strategy to adopt with parous women may be to avoid transfusing them, and this policy has been adopted by a number of transplant units including our own.

In most transplant units, previously non-transfused patients are transfused before transplantation. This practice is of course based on the finding, by Opelz and his colleagues in the early 1970s, of a superior graft survival rate in transfused compared with non-transfused patients[7]. Although a higher graft survival rate can be achieved with blood transfusions, a number of patients become sensitized to HLA antibodies, and some become highly sensitized. Because of this detrimental effect, a number of studies have been initiated to try to find a substitute for whole blood which will retain the beneficial effects while minimizing the sensitizing effects of transfusions. It is generally agreed that it is the leukocytes in the blood which cause sensitization and so some of the early studies examined the use of filtered, washed and frozen blood[8,9]. Filtered blood, from which all the leukocytes are removed, does not produce the 'transfusion effect'[9]. Washed blood, in which about 90% of the white cells are removed, can still cause sensitization[9]. Blood frozen by the centrifugal washing method, which removes all leukocytes, neither sensitizes nor produces a transfusion effect, whereas blood processed by agglomeration, which does not destroy all of the leukocytes, does produce a transfusion effect but also sensitizes a proportion of the patients[8]. From these studies, it is apparent that the leukocytes in the blood produce both the sensitizing and beneficial effects.

Some laboratories have investigated the use of HLA-matched blood (HLA-A,B matched with the patient), the rationale being that sensitization would be reduced. Although a reduction in sensitization was achieved, the effects of this type of transfusion on graft survival have been controversial. In one study, a beneficial effect was seen[10] while, in another, there was no advantage[11].

In the rat model, transfusion of platelets (which have class I histocompatibility antigens and not class II) can produce the beneficial

41

effects of blood in the absence of sensitization[12]. It was postulated that class I antigens (HLA-A, B, C in man) in the absence of class II (HLA-DR, DQ, DP in man) was not capable of producing a primary antibody response but could produce the 'transfusion effect'. Similar results have been seen in the monkey[13] but results in the dog have been equivocal[14,15]. Three studies of platelet transfusions in man have been carried out[16–18]. Two, by ourselves[16] and by Pallardo and his colleagues[17], showed no beneficial effect on graft survival while the study by Betuel and his colleagues[18] did show a beneficial effect. With regards to sensitization, we found that platelet suspensions contaminated with relatively few leukocytes could sensitize, whereas suspensions with no leukocytes did not. However, neither preparation could produce the 'transfusion effect'. The question of the use of platelet transfusions as a substitute for blood remains open.

Reducing the number of highly sensitized patients can best be achieved by increasing the survival rate of primary grafts, since a failed graft is the main cause in this group of patients. There are many factors which contribute to improved graft survival, such as HLA matching and the type of maintenance immunosuppression used. There is no doubt that the success rate of renal allografts has improved markedly in the last few years, and most people attribute this to the widespread use of cyclosporin. Even in this 'cyclosporin era', HLA matching (particularly for DR and B) can still improve graft survival[19,20].

Even with high survival rates, a significant number of grafts will fail and result in the accumulation of highly sensitized patients waiting for regrafts. Furthermore, pregraft blood transfusions are still given and some patients will become highly sensitized as a result. Therefore, investigation into ways of transplanting the highly sensitized patient are needed.

TRANSPLANTING THE HIGHLY SENSITIZED PATIENT

There are three ways of transplanting the highly sensitized patient:

1. Increasing the chances of finding a negative crossmatch donor.

2. Recognition that some highly sensitized patients have lym-

phocytotoxic antibodies which are not directed at HLA, and, in these patients, transplantation can be carried out in the presence of a positive crossmatch because the antibodies are not damaging to the graft.

3. In some patients who become highly sensitized, the level of antibody activity will decline with time. It has been suggested that only the latest sera (current sera), with no or low antibody reactivity, should be used for crossmatching and that the old highly reactive sera (peak sera) are clinically irrelevant.

1. Negative crossmatch donor

The chances of finding a kidney donor with a negative crossmatch (when peak and current sera are used) for a highly sensitized patient is remote, but can be improved by increasing the donor pool against which the sera are crossmatched. Several strategies have been developed to increase the chances of finding a crossmatch negative donor for these patients.

The United Kingdom Transplant Service (UKTS) set up a study (the SOS Scheme) in 1984 whereby sera from highly sensitized patients (> 85% panel reactive antibodies) from each participating centre are distributed to all other centres and crossmatched against all 'local' donors[21]. If a negative crossmatch is obtained, a kidney is sent to the appropriate recipient centre where additional sera from the patient are crossmatched, and, if these are negative, the transplant is performed. In the first two years of the Scheme, 232 patients have been entered and 83 (35%) have been transplanted. The 6-month graft survival rate for the whole group is 57%, and no difference is seen for first and second grafts (58% and 62%, respectively). The 13 third or fourth grafts have a 38% 6-month graft survival rate. It was noted that most grafts which failed did so within the first seven days after transplantation (20/36, 55%). Generally, no attempt was made to match the donor and recipient for HLA but the data do suggest that DR matching may influence graft survival; the 6-month survival rates of the grafts with 0 DR mismatches ($n = 25$) was 64%, 1 DR mismatches ($n = 34$) was 55%, and 2 DR mismatches ($n = 20$) was 50%.

43

Similar schemes to the UKTS SOS Scheme are operating within other organ-sharing organizations. For example, West Germany (HIT Study), Eurotransplant (the Highly Immunized File) and the South East Organ Procurement Foundation (ROP Study).

A second approach to increasing the chances of finding a negative crossmatch donor is to determine the HLA antigens against which the patient has *not* developed antibodies. These antigens together with the patient's own antigens will form the list of 'non-reactive antigens' or 'acceptable mismatches' for that patient. A donor who has any combination of these antigens should give a negative crossmatch. With this approach, sera from highly sensitized patients do not have to be shipped to other centres for crossmatching. Two methods have been used to determine a patient's acceptable mismatches. The first, which has been investigated by a number of laboratories, is to screen the sera against a large panel of cells and note the HLA antigens of the panel members to which the sera do not react[22,23]. The second, which is a novel scheme introduced by Claas and his colleagues[24], is to screen each serum against panel members selected so that only one HLA-A or -B antigen at a time is mismatched with the patient. In this study, sera from 73 highly sensitized patients were studied and, in 59, it was possible to define one or more acceptable mismatches. Thirty-four of these patients have been transplanted with a negative crossmatch kidney which, in addition, was DR compatible. The graft survival is 90% at 6 months and 86% at 12 months (22 patients at risk). This scheme has resulted in an extremely high graft survival rate and the authors have emphasized the importance of DR matching in this group of patients. This method has two drawbacks. Firstly, the tissue typing laboratory must have access to an extremely large pool of panel members. Secondly, it is very labour-intensive in that it takes one technician about two weeks to work-up one patient. Nevertheless, it is a method worth pursuing in a number of appropriately equipped laboratories.

A third approach is one which has been implemented by two groups[3,25] and is based on the supposition that sera from highly sensitized patients (reactive with $>70\%$ of a random cell panel) usually contain only one or two antibodies directed against the high-frequency public HLA antigens. By accurately characterizing the specificity of these cross-reactive antibodies, it is possible to predict

44

which donors are likely to give a negative crossmatch, and these would be the only ones crossmatched. This approach reduces the crossmatching workload of the laboratory and, at the same time, increases the chances of finding a negative crossmatch donor. This method has allowed a number of successful transplants to be performed in highly sensitized patients[25].

2. Recognition of non-HLA lymphocytotoxic antibodies

When the original crossmatch dogma was proposed it was assumed that all lymphocytotoxic antibodies were directed at HLA antigens. HLA antigens (class I and class II) are found on the endothelium of blood vessels in the kidney[26,27] and therefore it is reasonable to assume that pre-existing HLA antibodies in patients will cause immediate graft failure if they are directed at the donor's HLA antigens.

We now know that lymphocytotoxic antibodies with specificities other than HLA can be present in the sera of patients waiting for a renal transplant. The n.ain antibody specificities which we can now detect by lymphocytotoxicity are:

(i) HLA-A, -B and -C which react with both T and B lymphocytes,
(ii) HLA-DR, -DQ and -DP which react with B lymphocytes,
(iii) Autoantibodics against T and B lymphocytes,
(iv) Autoantibodies against B lymphocytes, and
(v) Non-autoreactive non-HLA antibodies which react with T and B lymphocytes or with B lymphocytes alone.

It is important to recognize the existence of these non-HLA antibodies since they often react with 100% of a random panel. Therefore, patients with this type of antibody will be thought of as highly sensitized although the antibody is not damaging to renal allografts; the evidence will be presented later. Autoantibodies can be distinguished from HLA antibodies by a number of characteristics, and these are summarized in Table 2.1 and discussed here.

45

TABLE 2.1   Some characteristics which distinguish autoantibodies from HLA antibodies

	Antibody specificity	
Characteristic	HLA	Auto
Antigenic stimuli	Preg/Tf/Tx	? Virus
Reactivity with normal lymphocytes	Yes	Yes
Reactivity with CLL cells	Yes	Yes/No
Reactivity with K562	No	Yes
Reactivity with autologous cells	No	Yes
Immunoglobulin class	IgG	IgM
Optimal temperature of reactivity	22–37°C	4°C
Inhibition by HLA monoclonal ab.	Yes	No

Antigenic stimuli

HLA amtibodies may occur after pregnancies, blood transfusion or renal transplantation, and only rarely do they appear 'spontaneously' although this has been documented[28]. Autoantibodies, on the other hand, usually appear 'spontaneously', not related to an obvious antigenic challenge, although there is some evidence that autoantibodies may appear after viral infections and, in particular, after cytomegalovirus infections[5,6].

Lymphocyte reactivity

HLA antibodies react with both normal and CLL lymphocytes since HLA antigens are present on both these cell types. Autoantibodies react with normal lymphocytes, where they can react with T and B lymphocytes[29] or with B lymphocytes alone[30]. Most autoantibodies do not react with, or only react weakly with, CLL cells[31]. Autoantibodies from most patients react with the cell line K562 whereas HLA antibodies do not[32]. By definition, autoantibodies react with the patient's own cells whereas HLA antibodies do not.

46

Immunoglobulin class

HLA antibodies are usually IgG, although some may be IgM particularly if produced while the patient is on immunosuppression[33]. Autoantibodies with few exceptions are IgM[34].

Optimal temperature for their detection

Autoantibodies react more strongly if the precomplement incubation step is performed at 4°C than at room temperature[35], although they can be reactive at 37°C[36]. HLA antibodies react well at all precomplement incubation temperatures.

Cytotoxicity inhibition by monoclonal antibodies

The cytotoxic reactivity of HLA antibodies is inhibited by prior incubation of the target cells with mouse monoclonal antibodies to the appropriate monomorphic determinants of HLA class I (A, B, C), HLA-DR, and HLA-DQ[34,37]. The cytotoxicity of autoantibodies is not inhibited by these monoclonal antibodies.

The specificity of the target antigen to which autoantibodies react is largely unknown, although there is evidence that the B cell autoantibody is directed at IgM[38]. Autoantibodies which occur in patients with systemic lupus erythematosus may be directed at β_2-microglobulin[39].

The incidence of autoantibodies in a dialysis population has been reported to be as high as 42%[40], although most laboratories find a considerably lower incidence[41]. We have found that autoantibodies occur more often in post-transplant than in pregraft sera, and, in these sera, there is often a mixture of autoantibodies and HLA antibodies.

The benign nature of autoantibodies was first shown in 1976 by the reports of successful transplantation of cadaver grafts[42] and a living related donor graft[43] in the presence of a T and B cell crossmatch due to these antibodies. There is now overwhelming evidence that autoantibodies, whether they react with T and B lymphocytes or with

47

B lymphocytes only, are not damaging to renal allograft, even when they react with the donor's lymphocytes[29,44]. Our most recent results of cadaver transplants in highly sensitized patients with a positive crossmatch due to autoantibodies are shown in Table 2.2. In recipients

TABLE 2.2   The outcome of cadaver grafts transplanted in highly sensitized patients in Oxford with a T and B cell positive or B cell positive crossmatch due to autoantibodies, or with a negative crossmatch

	Crossmatch			% Graft survival (months)			
Graft no.	T	B	No.	1	3	6	12
First	+	+	18	78	72	72	60
First	−	+	9	100	89	89	89
First	−	−	7	71	57	57	43
Regraft	+	+	20	75	70	65	65
Regraft	−	+	7	71	57	43	43
Regraft	−	−	7	71	71	71	57

of a first graft, a very high success rate is seen in the B cell positive crossmatch transplants, and, in fact, the highly sensitized patients with a negative crossmatch have the lowest survival rate. However, the survival rates in the three groups are not significantly different. Eight living related donor grafts have also been performed with a positive crossmatch due to autoantibodies and the results are summarized in Table 2.3. Only one of these grafts has failed (TW) and this was due to chronic rejection. Our data are certainly consistent with the view that autoantibodies are clinically irrelevant to graft outcome.

3. Peak sera positive, current sera negative (P + C −) crossmatch

In some patients who become highly sensitized, the level of their antibody activity may decline with time to a lower level or even disappear altogether. Normally, such patients are still difficult to transplant since it has been the standard procedure to use a number of sera for crossmatching, including the old sera with the peak antibody reactivity.

TABLE 2.3 Transplantation of living related donor grafts in highly sensitized recipients in Oxford with a positive T and B cell crossmatch due to autoantibodies

Patient	Graft no.	No. shared haplotypes	XM at Tx	Outcome	Follow-up (months)
JF	1	2	+	Success	114
TW	3	1	−	Failed	72
ST	1	2	+	Success	77
MF	2	2	−	Success	48
MS	1	1	+	Success	51
WS	1	2	+	Success	43
TA	1	1	+	Success	30
RR	1	2	+	Success	6

However, this practice was seriously questioned by Cardella and his colleagues from Toronto[45] who suggested that the peak sera may not be clinically relevant for crossmatching. This conclusion was based on their finding of successful transplant outcome in a number of patients with a P + C− crossmatch with their donors. This study caused tremendous interest for, if it could be confirmed, many patients considered not transplantable using conventional crossmatch protocols may be able to receive a successful transplant. Confirmation of this pioneering work soon appeared in the literature[46–48,34]. These studies have caused such an impact on crossmatching policies that now a number of transplant units discard sera that are six or 12 months old, and only crossmatch the recently collected sera!

In the majority of patients where a P + C− crossmatch transplant has been performed, the level of antibody activity in the patients has fallen 'naturally' with time, but, in some patients, an active attempt has been made to remove the antibody in patients who have shown persistently high levels of antibodies. Taube and his colleagues in London first reported the removal of HLA antibodies and prevention of their resynthesis by treating patients with a combination of plasmapheresis, cyclophosphamide and prednisolone[49]. In their first report of five patients treated while waiting for regrafts, four were successfully transplanted and one died with a poorly-functioning graft. The authors admitted that although the method was successful in removing HLA antibodies, it should be reserved for patients with overwhelming

49

clinical or social reasons for transplantation because of the significant morbidity associated with the treatment. Plasmapheresis has also been used successfully by other groups[50]. More recently, Taube's group[51] have used extracorporeal immunoadsorption on protein A columns to remove IgG HLA antibodies. This protocol was carried out in four patients, three of whom were subsequently successfully transplanted. In spite of the successes the authors believe that not all patients are suited for the treatment and only those with one main HLA antibody specificity are likely to benefit (K. Welsh, personal communication). The supposition is that a highly reactive serum contains one main HLA specificity to a 'private' epitope and the rest of the reactivity is due to the weaker crossreactive antibodies. Treatment by plasmapheresis or immunoadsorption is thought to remove the crossreactive antibodies, and a kidney is found which does not have the HLA antigen to which the main specificity is directed. Antithymocyte globulin (ATG) is given prophylactically in these patients and this may be important is securing a successful graft outcome.

There is no doubt that transplants with a $P + C -$ crossmatch due to HLA can be successfully carried out. However, caution should be exercised when considering such a transplant since a number of grafts have suffered immediate failure, suggesting that the optimal conditions for performing such transplants have not been fully worked out. Some of the key questions which are still being examined and which need to be answered are:

(i) Is there a minimum time interval between the last positive serum and the time of transplantation?

(ii) Are certain patients at a higher risk than others? For example, recipients of a regraft compared with those of a first graft.

(iii) Is an HLA well-matched graft necessary, and should previous mismatched HLA antigens be avoided in regrafts?

(iv) Are there prognostic indicators which can predict which grafts are likely to be successful and which might fail?

The minimum time interval between the last serum giving a positive crossmatch and transplantation has varied from 1 month[52] to 12 months[34] and there does not appear to be any agreement. As mentioned previously, a number of laboratories now do not crossmatch sera which is more than 6–12 months old.

50

Regrafts performed in the presence of a P + C − crossmatch have a lower success rate than first grafts, although Cardella and his group showed that the success rate was still the same as that seen in regrafts in patients with a negative crossmatch using all sera[52]. Therefore, the lower success rate may be due to the fact that patients who have rejected a previous graft are immunological high-risk patients and this is not affected by whether they receive a P + C − or a P − C − regraft.

In most studies reported, there has been no attempt to find an HLA well-matched graft. We[34] and others[46] have avoided previous HLA mismatched antigens in regrafts, although this policy is by no means practised by all units[34]. Perhaps attention should be paid to better HLA matching for regrafts, particularly for DR antigens, since there is some evidence (previously discussed) that this may increase the likelihood for success in highly sensitized patients.

A significant proportion of P + C − crossmatch grafts fail soon after transplantation and it would be extremely useful if such an occurrence could be predicted before transplantation. With this aim in mind, we examined the immunoglobulin class of the HLA antibody causing the positive crossmatch and found that those due to an IgG antibody invariably failed, and a successful outcome was seen only if the antibody causing the positive crossmatch was an IgM[34]. We have extended this initial retrospective study and the current data are shown in Table 2.4. The data show that only one patient with an IgG antibody has been successfully transplanted and it is perhaps interesting to note that this patient received ATG prophylactically when it was realised that the antibody was IgG HLA class I. Although the numbers studied are small, the conclusion from our finding is that a successful graft with a P + C − crossmatch is likely only if the antibody is IgM.

TABLE 2.4   Peak serum positive, current serum negative crossmatch transplants performed in Oxford. A correlation between the immunoglobulin (Ig) class of the antibody and graft outcome

Ig class	No. patients	Successful at 6 months
Igm	15	10 (67%)
IgG	9	1 (11%)

Reed and her colleagues[53] have suggested that the presence of anti-idiotypic antibodies in the current serum directed against the HLA specificity present in the peak reactive serum may be indicative of a successful outcome. These authors found that all nine patients with a successful $P + C-$ crossmatch graft had anti-idiotypic antibodies, whereas only one of nine patients whose grafts failed had anti-idiotypic antibodies.

Although a number of 'unknowns' still exist, there is no doubt that successful transplantation can be carried out with a $P + C-$ crossmatch due to HLA class I antibodies.

CROSSMATCHING IN HIGHLY SENSITIZED PATIENTS

The crossmatch protocol varies markedly from one laboratory to another, not just for highly sensitized patients, but for all patients. We have based our crossmatch protocol for highly sensitized patients on the premise that IgM antibodies, whether directed against HLA or non-HLA antigens, are not damaging to renal allografts (and the data to support this hypothesis have been discussed). In addition, we insist on a completely negative crossmatch from sera collected during the 12 months prior to transplantation. Our protocol is as follows:

(i) The highest reactive serum from all highly sensitized patients are dispensed into plates (local SOS plates) and frozen at $-80°C$.

(ii) A selection of up to 10 highly reactive sera from each highly sensitized patient are dispensed into plates, such that each patient has individual plates.
  Note: Sera known to have only autoantibodies are not included in these plates.

(iii) The local SOS plate is crossmatched against the unseparated spleen cells of all local donors. The sera are tested (a) untreated, (b) after the addition of dithiothreitol (DTT) which destroys the IgM molecule, and (c) after the addition of phosphate buffered saline (PBS) as a control.

(iv) A patient who gives a negative crossmatch with either untreated or DTT-treated serum is recrossmatched against the donor's T cells using their individual trays; again tested untreated, with DTT and with PBS.

(v) A patient is considered for transplantation under one of two conditions.

    (a) All untreated (and treated) sera give a negative crossmatch.

    (b) Sera collected over the last 12 months give a negative crossmatch when untreated, even if the older sera give a positive crossmatch when untreated, but this must be negative after DTT treatment.

CONCLUSIONS

The outlook for the highly sensitized patient has certainly changed (for the better) during the last decade. Blood transfusions (given with care), HLA matching (particularly for the DR and B antigens), more potent immunosuppression, to name a few of the measurable factors, have led to a marked improvement in the success rate of primary renal allografts and a concomitant decrease in the number of patients becoming highly sensitized.

There is no doubt that the original dogma, that a transplant should not be performed in the presence of a positive lymphocytotoxic crossmatch, is no longer tenable. This is because: firstly, the realization that the antibodies in some patients are not directed at HLA and these are not damaging to renal allografts; and secondly, the finding that it may only be necessary to crossmatch the 'current' sera. Both of these findings have dramatically changed our understanding of lymphocytotoxic antibodies and their relevance in the crossmatch test. As a result, the transplantation prospects of the highly sensitized patient has markedly improved.

REFERENCES

1. Terasaki, P. I., Marchioro, T. L. and Starzl, T. E. (eds.) (1965). Sero-typing of human lymphocyte antigens: Preliminary trials on long-term kidney homograft survivors. *Histocompatibility Testing*, pp. 83–96. (Washington, D.C.: National Academy of Science)

2. Williams, G. M., Hume, D.M., Hudson, R.P., Morris, P.J., Kano, K. and Milgrom, F. (1968). 'Hyperacute' renal-homograft rejection in man. *N. Engl. J. Med.*, **279**, 611-618

3. Oldfather, J. W., Anderson, C. B., Phelan, D. L., Cross, D. E., Luger, A. M. and Rodey, G. E. (1986). Prediction of crossmatch outcome in highly sensitized dialysis patients based on the identification of serum HLA antibodies. *Transplantation*, **42**, 267-270

4. Opelz, G., Graver, B., Mickey, M. R. and Terasaki, P. I. (1981). Lymphocytotoxic antibody responses to transfusions in potential kidney transplant recipients. *Transplantation*, **32**, 177-183

5. Jeannet, M. and Stalder, H. (1978). Lymphocytotoxic antibodies in spontaneous cytomegalovirus infection. *Lancet*, **1**, 509

6. MacLeod, A. M., Kurtz, J., Chapman, J. R., Ting, A. and Morris, P. J. (1987). Autolymphocytotoxins and virus infection in renal transplantation. *Transplant. Proc.*, **19**, 901

7. Opelz, G., Sengar, D. P. S., Mickey, M. R. and Terasaki, P. I. (1973). Effect of blood transfusions on subsequent kidney transplants. *Transplant. Proc.*, **5**, 253-259

8. Fuller, T. C., Delmonico, F. L., Cosimi, A. B., Huggins, C. E., King, M. and Russell, P. S. (1977). Effects of various types of RBC transfusions on HLA alloimmunization and renal allograft survival. *Transplant. Proc.*, **9**, 117-119

9. Persijn, G. G., Cohen, B., Lansbergen, Q. and Van Rood, J. J. (1979). Retrospective and prospective studies on the effect of blood transfusions in renal transplantation in the Netherlands. *Transplantation*, **28**, 396-401

10. Nube, M. J., Persijn, G. G., Van Es, A., Kalff, M. W., De Graeff, J. and Van Rood, J. J. (1983). Beneficial effect of HLA-A and B matched pretransplant blood transfusions on primary cadaveric kidney graft survival. *Transplantation*, **35**, 556-561

11. Albert, E. D., Scholz, S., Meixner, U. and Land, W. (1981). HLA-A, B matching of pretransplant blood transfusion is associated with poor graft survival. *Transplant. Proc.*, **13**, 175-177

12. Welsh, K. I., Burgos, H. and Batchelor, J. R. (1977). The immune response to allogeneic rat platelets; Ag-B antigens in matrix form lacking Ia. *Eur. J. Immunol.*, **7**, 267-272

13. Borleffs, J. C. C., Neuhaus, P., Van Rood, J. J. and Balner, H. (1982). Platelet transfusions improve kidney allograft survival in rhesus monkeys without inducing cytotoxic antibodies. *Lancet*, **1**, 1117-1118

14. Bijnen, A. B., Heineman, E., Marquet, R. L., Niessen, G. J. C. M., Obertop, H., Tank, B. and Jeekel, J. (1984). Lack of beneficial effect of thrombocyte transfusions on kidney graft survival in dogs. *Transplantation*, **37**, 213-214

15. Errett, L. E., Allen, N., Deierhoi, M. H., Denton, T. G., Wood, R. F. M. and Morris, P. J. (1985). The effect of platelet transfusions on renal allograft survival and sensitisation in dogs. *Tissue Antigens*, **25**, 28-32

16. Chapman, J. R., Ting, A., Fisher, M., Carter, N. P. and Morris, P. J. (1986). Failure of platelet transfusion to improve human renal allograft survival. *Transplantation*, **41**, 468-473

17. Pallardo, L. M., Montoro, J., Moll, J. M., Sanchez, J., Sóler, M. A., Marty, M. and Cruz, J. M. (1985). Platelet transfusions do not improve cadaveric renal allograft survival. *Transplant. Proc.*, **17**, 2338-2339

18. Betuel, H., Cantarovitch, D., Robert, F., Gebuhrer, L., Touraine, J. L., Dubernard, J. M. and Traeger, J. (1985). Platelet transfusions preparative for kidney transplantation. *Transplant. Proc.*, **17**, 2335–2337

19. Opelz, G. for the Collaborative Transplant Study (1987). Effect of HLA matching in 10,000 cyclosporine-treated cadaver kidney transplants. *Transplant. Proc.*, **19**, 641–646

20. Ting, A. and Morris, P. J. (1987). HLA matching in transfused, cyclosporine-treated patients at Oxford. In Terasaki, P. I. (ed.) *Clinical Transplants 1987*. (Los Angeles, California: UCLA Tissue Typing Laboratory) pp. 235–238

21. Bradley, B. A., Klouda, P. T., Ray, T. C. and Gore, S. M. (1985). Negative crossmatch selection of kidneys for highly sensitized patients. *Transplant. Proc.*, **17**, 2465–2466

22. Mickey, M. R., Ayoub, G. and Terasaki, P. I. (1982). Prediction of negative crossmatch: An aid for cost-effective kidney sharing. *Transplant. Proc.*, **14**, 279–281

23. Klouda, P. T., Ray, T. C., Bowerman, P. and Bradley, B. A. (1985). The prediction of a negative crossmatch in highly sensitized patients. *Transplant. Proc.*, **17**, 2467–2468

24. Claas, F. H. J. and van Rood, J. J. (1988). The hyperimmunized patient: from sensitization toward transplantation. *Transplant. Int.*, **1**, 53–57

25. Delmonico, F. L., Fuller, A., Cosimi, A. B., Tolkoff-Rubin, N., Russell, P. S., Rodney, G. E. and Fuller, T. C. (1983). New approaches to donor crossmatching and successful transplantation of highly sensitized patients. *Transplantation*, **36**, 629–633

26. Daar, A. S., Fuggle, S. V., Fabre, J. W., Ting, A. and Morris, P. J. (1984). The detailed distribution of HLA-A, B, C antigens in normal human organs. *Transplantation*, **38**, 287–292

27. Daar, A. S., Fuggle, S. V., Fabre, J. W., Ting, A. and Morris, P. J. (1984). The detailed distribution of MHC class II antigens in normal human organs. *Transplantation*, **38**, 293–298

28. Tongio, M. M. and Mayer, S. (1985). Naturally occurring HLA antibodies. *Transplant. Clin. Immunol.*, **17**, 45–56

29. Ting, A. and Morris, P. J. (1983). Successful transplantation with a positive T and B cell crossmatch due to autoreactive antibodies. *Tissue Antigens*, **21**, 219–226

30. Reekers, P., Lucassen-Hermans, R., Koene, R. A. P. and Kunst, V. A. J. M. (1977). Autolymphocytotoxic antibodies and kidney transplantation. *Lancet*, **1**, 1063–1064

31. Ting, A. and Morris, P. J. (1978). Reactivity of autolymphocytotoxic antibodies from dialysis patients with lymphocytes from chronic lymphocytic leukemia (CLL) patients. *Transplantation*, **25**, 31–33

32. Deierhoi, M. H., Ting, A. and Morris, P. J. (1984). Reactivity of lymphocyte cytotoxic autoantibodies from renal patients with cell line K562. *Transplantation*, **38**, 557–558

33. Stocker, J. W., McKenzie, I. F. C. and Morris, P. J. (1969). IgM activity in human lymphocytotoxic sera after renal transplantation. *Nature (London)*, **222**, 483–484

34. Chapman, J. R., Taylor, C. J., Ting, A. and Morris, P. J. (1986). Immunoglobulin class and specificity of antibodies causing positive T cell crossmatches: Relationship to renal transplant outcome. *Transplantation*, **42**, 608–613

35. Park, M. S., Terasaki, P. I. and Bernocco, D. (1977). Autoantibody against B lymphocytes. *Lancet*, **2**, 465–467
36. Deierhoi, M. H., Ting, A. and Morris, P. J. (1983). Successful renal transplantation despite warm B cell antibodies. *Transplantation*, **36**, 207–209
37. Taylor, C. J., Chapman, J. R., Fuggle, S. V., Ting, A. and Morris, P. J. (1987). A positive B cell crossmatch due to IgG anti-HLA-DQ antibody present at the time of transplantation in a successful renal allograft. *Tissue Antigens*, **30**, 104–112
38. Cicciarelli, J. C., Chia, D., Terasaki, P. I., Barnett, E. V. and Shirahama, S. (1980). Human IgM anti-IgM cytotoxin for B lymphocytes. *Tissue Antigens*, **15**, 275–282
39. Revillard, J. P., Vincent, C. and Rivera, S. (1979). Anti-β_2-microglobulin lymphocytotoxic autoantibodies in systemic lupus erythematosus. *J. Immunol.*, **122**, 614–618
40. Lobo, P. I. (1981). Nature of autolymphocytotoxins present in renal hemodialysis patients. Their possible role in controlling alloantibody formation. *Transplantation*, **32**, 233–237
41. Ettenger, R. B., Jordan, S. and Fine, R. N. (1981). Autolymphocytotoxic antibodies in patients on dialysis awaiting renal transplantation. *Transplantation*, **32**, 248–251
42. Cross, D. E., Greiner, R. and Whittier, F. C. (1976). Importance of the autocontrol crossmatch in human renal transplantation. *Transplantation*, **21**, 307–311
43. Stastny, P. and Austin, C. L. (1976). Successful kidney transplant in patient with positive crossmatch due to autoantibodies. *Transplantation*, **21**, 399–402
44. Ettenger, R. B., Jordan, S. C. and Fine, R. N. (1983). Cadaver renal transplant outcome in recipients with autolymphocytotoxic antibodies. *Transplantation*, **35**, 429–431
45. Cardella, C. J., Falk, J. A., Nicholson, M. J., Harding, M. and Cook, G. T. (1982). Successful renal transplantation in patients with T-cell reactivity to donor. *Lancet*, **2**, 1240–1243
46. Mates, A. J., Nehlsen-Cannarella, S., Tellis, V. A., Kuemmel, P., Soberman, R. and Veith, F. J. (1984). Successful kidney transplantation with current-sera-negative/historical-sera-positive T cell crossmatch. *Transplantation*, **37**, 111–112
47. Fuller, T. C., Forbes, J. B. and Delmonico F. L. (1985). Renal transplantation with a positive historical donor crossmatch. *Transplant. Proc.*, **17**, 113–114
48. Goeken, N. E. and the Clinical Affairs Committee (1985). Outcome of renal transplantation following a positive cross-match with historical sera: The ASHI survey. *Human Immunol.*, **14**, 77–85
49. Taube, D. H., Williams, D. G., Cameron, J. S., Bewick, M., Ogg, C. S., Rudge, C. J., Welsh, K. I., Kennedy, L. A. and Thick, M. G. (1984). Renal transplantation after removal and prevention of resynthesis of HLA antibodies. *Lancet*, **1**, 824–826
50. Hillebrand, G., Castro, L. A., Samtleben, W., Albert, E., Scholz, S., Illner, W. D., Land, W. and Gurland, H. J. (1985). Removal of preformed cytotoxic antibodies in highly sensitized patients using plasma exchange and immunosuppressive therapy, azathioprine, or cyclosporine prior to renal transplantation. *Transplant. Proc.*, **17**, 2501–2504
51. Palmer, A., Taube, D., Welsh, K., Brynger, H., Delin, K., Gjorstrup, P., Konar,

J. and Soderstrom, T. (1987). Extracorporeal immunoadsorption of anti-HLA antibodies; Preliminary clinical experience. *Transplant. Proc.*, **19**, 3750–3751.
52. Cardella, C. J., Falk, J. A., Halloran, P., Robinette, M., Arbus, G. and Bear, R. (1985). Renal transplantation in patients with a positive crossmatch on non-current sera: Long-term follow-up. *Transplant. Proc.*, **17**, 626–627
53. Reed, E., Hardy, M., Benvenitsky, A., Lattes, C., Brensilver, J., McCabe, R., Reemstma, K., King, D. W. and Suciu-Foca, N. (1987). Effect of antiidiotypic antibodies to HLA on graft survival in renal allograft recipients. *N. Engl. J. Med.*, **316**, 1450–1455

3
TISSUE TYPING POLICY

V. C. JOYSEY

What is tissue typing and how might it influence policy in relation to kidney transplantation? To answer these questions, some relationships between tissue matching, graft survival and function will be considered. Present policy and whether it could be improved will then be discussed.

Tissue type is the colloquial name for the blood group antigens of the nucleated cells. These are most easily demonstrated on the leukocytes and therefore they are known as the human leukocyte antigens, HLA. The HLA system of man is the homologue of the H2 system of the mouse and these are part of the major histocompatibility system, MHS, which is present in all mammals and is very complex in all species in which it has been studied. When skin grafts are performed between mice, matching of the H2 antigens between donor and recipient has been found to prolong survival of the grafts[1].

The HLA system is controlled by a number of closely linked complex loci on chromosome 6 that define several different categories of biologically important antigenic markers (Figure 3.1). Among these are the class 1 antigens – HLA-A, HLA-B and HLA-CW which are present on all nucleated cells of the body and can be regarded as the body's antigenic 'uniform' by which it identifies self from not-self, and the class 2 antigens – HLA-DR, HLA-DP and HLA-DQ which are present on B lymphocytes, Kupffer cells and activated T cells, and are involved in cell-to-cell communication.

At each HLA locus there is a large number of alternative alleles which define different antigens (Table 3.1).

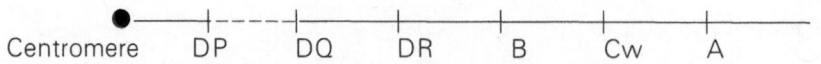

Centromere   DP   DQ   DR   B   Cw   A

FIGURE 3.1   Simplified diagram of the arrangement of loci defining HLA antigens in the HLA region of chromosome 6

Each (normal) individual is diploid and therefore can have no more than 2 antigens coded by any one locus. Each individual has two chromosome 6 and, in the production of germ cells, at meiosis, these separate. Each chromosome 6 carries a closely linked group of HLA markers (HLA-A, B, Cw, DR, DQ and DP) which is known as a haplotype: that is, the haploid expression of the HLA type. The antigens of one haplotype are conveyed as a unit *en bloc* to the offspring. Each parent has two haplotypes and, in the absence of crossing over (which is rare), these can combine to produce only 4 combinations of HLA antigens in the offspring (Table 3.2). This gives a $\frac{1}{4}$ possibility of any two full siblings being HLA identical, a $\frac{1}{2}$ chance of them sharing one haplotype and a $\frac{1}{4}$ chance of them differing at both haplotypes. Because they share two whole haplotypes, HLA identical siblings are identical on the HLA markers that we cannot yet detect. This is important in transplantation from a family donor who may share one or two HLA haplotypes with the recipient.

The different HLA-A, B, C and DR antigens are not randomly arranged on the haplotypes; some combinations are very much more common than others. This is almost certainly because there are biological advantages in having certain combinations of antigens. Some common haplotypes in the UK are HLA-A1, B8, DR3 / HLA-A3, B7, DR2 / HLA-A2, B12, DR4. Because some haplotypes are common, matching of the antigens of a donor and recipient for a kidney graft is often much easier than the multiplicity of HLA antigens would suggest.

The test usually used to define class 1 and class 2 antigens before transplant is based on a lymphocytotoxic test, i.e. aliquots of anti-HLA antisera of defined specificity are incubated with live lymphocytes and rabbit serum (complement). If the antibody combines with the lymphocytes, the cells are killed and the percentage cell death is monitored, usually by staining. The test is theoretically very easy

TABLE 3.1   HLA specificities recognized in 1987

HLA-A
A1 / A2 / A3 / A9(A23)(A24) / A10(A25)(A26)(Aw34)(Aw66) / A11 /
Aw19(A29)(A30)(A31)(A32)(Aw33)(Aw74) / A28(Aw68)(Aw69) / Aw36 /
Aw43

HLA-B
B5(B51)(Bw52) / B7 / B8 / B12(B44)(B45) / B13 / B14(Bw64)(Bw65) /
B15(Bw62)(Bw63)(Bw75)(Bw76)(Bw77) / B16(B38)(B39) /
B17(Bw57)(Bw58) / B18 / B21(B49)(Bw50) / Bw22(Bw54)(Bw55)(Bw56) /
B27 / B35 / B37 / B40(Bw60)(Bw61) / Bw41 / Bw42 /Bw46 /Bw47 /
Bw48 / Bw53 / Bw59 / Bw67 / Bw70(Bw71)(Bw72) / Bw73

HLA-C
Cw1 / Cw2 / Cw3(Cw9)(Cw10) / Cw4 / Cw5 / Cw6 / Cw7 / Cw8 / Cw11

HLA-D
Dw1 / Dw2 / Dw3 / Dw4 / Dw5 / Dw6(Dw18)(Dw19) / Dw7(Dw11)
(Dw17) / Dw8 / Dw9 / Dw10 / Dw12 / Dw13 / Dw14 / Dw15 / Dw16 /
Dw20 / Dw21 / Dw22 /Dw23 / Dw24 / Dw25 / Dw26

HLA-DR
DR1 / DR2(DRw15)(DRw16) / DR3(DRw17)(DRw18) / DR4 / DR5
(DRw11)(DRw12) / DRw6(DRw13)(DRw14) / DR7 / DRw8 / DR9 /
DRw10 / DRw52 / DRw53

HLA-DQ
DQw1(DQw5)(DQw6) / DQw2 / DQw3(DQw7)(DQw8)(DQw9) / DQw4

HLA-DP
DPw1 / DPw2 / DPw3 / DPw4 / DPw5 / DPw6

Antigens in parentheses are subspecificities of the preceding broad specificity. Some combinations of antigens are common, e.g. A2, B12, DR4, so it is less difficult to get well-matched grafts than the multiplicity of antigens might suggest

but, unless performed meticulously, it is also very easy to get the wrong answer! In addition, the reagents available, especially for class 2 antigen definition, show cross reactivity and therefore a large number of test sera are needed to give a 'majority verdict'. However, in the hands of experienced workers, using well-authenticated sera, good repeatable results can be obtained. Definition of class 1 antigens, HLA-A, B and CW, is usually good as excellent sera are available. Unfortunately, definition of some DR antigens is still difficult and liable to error, e.g. DRw6, as the sera available are usually of mixed

TABLE 3.2   Inheritance of HLA antigens

	Father		**Mother**
Haplotype	a. A1, B8, DR3	Haplotype	c. A3, B7, DR2
	b. A2, B12, DR4		d. A11, Bw22, DRw8

Offspring

1. Haplotype a. A1, B8, DR3
            c. A3, B7, DR2
2. Haplotype a. A1, B8, DR3
            d. A11, Bw22, DRw8
3. Haplotype b. A2, B12, DR4
            c. A3, B7, DR2
4. Haplotype b. A2, B12, DR4
            d. All, Bw22, DRw8

specificity. The definition of DR by the cytotoxic test has improved steadily in UK laboratories over the last ten years. However, it is not yet perfect, particularly in potential kidney graft recipients who are notoriously difficult to type as antigens may be 'missed' because of low reactivity of the cells. DQ and DP typing is not yet widely carried out by serological tests.

HLA-D antigens were originally defined by mixed leukocyte culture (MLC). In this test, the class 2 antigenic difference between cells of two individuals is defined by the biological response of the cells themselves. Lymphocytes of 2 people are co-cultured, after the cells of one of the individuals, the stimulator, have been rendered incapable of DNA synthesis by means of X-irradiation. The cells of the second participant, the responder, go into DNA synthesis in response to the class 2 antigens present in the stimulator and absent from the responder. After several days, the amount of DNA synthesis is monitored by pulsing the culture with tritiated thymidine.

Thymidine incorporation is proportional to DNA synthesis, which is a reflection of the class 2 antigenic disparity between the stimulator and the responder as recognized by the responder lymphocytes. Thymidine incorporation can be maximal, intermediate or background, depending on whether the responder cells recognize two, one or zero HLA-D antigens as foreign. Cells which are known to be homozygous for HLA-D can be used to HLA-D 'type' unknown cells in MLC by using each of them in turn as stimulator and responder in combination with the other. This technique has enabled the definition of at least 24 HLA-D antigens. The HLA-D antigens were originally thought to be the same as the antigens detectable by lymphocytotoxic tests on B cells. There is a considerable degree of association, but it was soon realized that the serological test and MLC were not detecting the same determinants and therefore the serologically defined antigens were called HLA-DR, i.e. D related. It is likely that the discrimination of antigenic definition by the lymphocytes is finer than that by the cytotoxic test. However, because of the time taken to carry out MLC tests, it is impracticable to use this technique for prospective antigen matching, except in the case of living related donors. Within a family, the potential donor who is least stimulatory to the recipient in MLC is likely to constitute the best donor.

A new method of defining HLA-DR antigens is now available by restriction fragment length polymorphism studies (RFLP). This method is more accurate than the cytotoxic test but takes several days and is therefore not yet useful for prospective cadaver kidney donor typing. However, it can be used now as an aid to definition of recipient HLA-DR groups on recipients who have been difficult to type. Clearly, antigen definition is crucial if it is to be used to select donors for kidney graft recipients.

From the viewpoint of a kidney transplant patient, does the tissue matching that we can carry out with our present serological tests matter? In order to answer this question, it is necessary to review results of kidney transplants in relation to donor and recipient red cell ABO groups, lymphocytotoxic crossmatching, and HLA-A, B and DR matching.

ABO COMPATIBILITY

If a kidney is transplanted into an ABO incompatible recipient, it is usually hyperacutely rejected. The anti-A and/or anti-B in the serum of the recipient combines with the appropriate A or B antigen present on donor tissue cells and death of the kidney is often rapid. For this reason, kidney transplantation is usually only performed between ABO compatible donors and recipients.

Breimer and colleagues found that 14 A2 kidneys grafted into group O recipients were not hyperacutely rejected[2]. When treated with conventional immunosuppression, ten of these had 'long term' function, the longest surviving 'over 6 years'. However, of 6 further transplants treated with cyclosporin A, none had long-term function. Rydberg[3], Welsh[4], Shapira[5] and their colleagues reported grafting of kidneys from A2 donors into ABO incompatible recipients without hyeracute rejection but some needed vigorous immunosuppressive therapy to retain their kidney. The Guys Hospital group have suggested that further investigations are needed before A2 donors are used widely for incompatible recipients[4].

Cook and colleagues studied the survival of 25 cadaver donor ABO-incompatible grafts which had been carried out unintentionally[6]. Of these, only one survived longer than 1 year (4% survival), substantiating the current practice of seeking ABO compatibility. In the account that follows, ABO compatibility was, as far as is known, present in all grafts.

CROSSMATCH TESTS

If anti-HLA antibody is present in the serum of a kidney recipient to an HLA antigen of the donor, hyperacute rejection normally ensues. To try to avoid this, a cytotoxic crossmatch of the serum of the graft recipient against the lymphocytes of the potential donor is carried out before transplant. If the crossmatch is positive, i.e. the recipient serum kills potential donor cells, the transplant is not performed. This is true if the antibody is IgG of anti-HLA specificity. However, IgM autoantibody also causes cytotoxicity under the normal test conditions but is believed to be of no clinical significance to graft survival[7]. It is possible to discriminate between these two types of antibody by carrying out two crossmatch tests in parallel, one normal test and the other in the presence of dithiothreitol (DTT). DTT cleaves IgM and ablates the reaction of the antibody. Therefore, if the DTT crossmatch test is negative, the normal positive crossmatch test of the same serum sample can be ignored.

Serum samples of patients awaiting transplant are regularly screened by the cytotoxic test against a panel of lymphocytes of normal individuals in order to define the strength, specificity and frequency of reaction of antibodies in the patients' sera. After the patient has been stimulated by HLA antigens, as occurs during pregnancy, blood transfusion and organ transplant, the anti-HLA antibody strength and frequency of reaction against the panel may rise, but, in the absence of stimulus, the antibody may decline with time. The 'peak' serum sample, i.e. that with the highest titre and greatest frequency of reaction may give a positive crossmatch while the current serum sample gives a negative crossmatch. What policy should be followed?

The work of Falk[8] and Kerman[9] and colleagues shows that if the current serum gives a negative crossmatch with the donor, even though a historical serum sample of the patient gives a positive crossmatch, then survival for first grafts may be not detectably different from those with a historical negative and current negative crossmatch result. These studies did not address whether the antibody causing the historical positive crossmatch was autoantibody or alloantibody. In four regrafts, Kerman and colleagues noted that the survival of grafts with historical positive and current negative crossmatches was poor[9], suggesting that anti-HLA antibody might have been responsible for graft failure. Many transplant centres now ignore a historical positive crossmatch if the crossmatch with current serum is negative. The sensitivity of the crossmatch is important. An IgG anti-HLA antibody which causes a weak positive reaction is capable of causing hyperacute rejection but this will not be detected if an insensitive test is used.

OVERALL TRANSPLANT SURVIVAL

Survival of kidney transplants is often expressed in the form of actuarial curves, which show the grafts surviving at times after transplant as a percentage of the total grafts carried out. Examination of the figures illustrating this chapter will demonstrate that the greatest loss of kidney grafts occurs during the first 3 months after transplant.

A large number of factors are relevant to survival of an allografted kidney, e.g. blood transfusion prior to grafting, presence of cytotoxic antibody in the recipient, the number of the allograft, i.e., 1st, 2nd or 3rd graft, the age, race of both the donor and recipient, ischaemic time of the donor kidney, original disease of the recipient, and method of preservation of the kidney, as well as the more obvious factors, such as the skill of the surgeons and clinical management of the immunosuppression of the patient. The percentage graft survival differs widely between different transplant centres: the so called 'centre effect'. Multicentre studies inevitably have a larger background variability than small single-centre investigations. Some large series, such as the Collaborative Transplant Study, however, have a common set of anti-HLA sera to be used by participants from different centres and this limits one of the causes of variability. Data on large numbers of transplants from diverse centres can only be obtained by multicentre studies, but are essential for the valid evaluation of factors relevant to long-term function of transplanted kidneys.

Over the last two decades, overall transplant survival has greatly improved with advances in immunosuppressive techniques and with experience gained by the transplant teams. The relevance of different factors, e.g. HLA compatibility, may vary with different immunosuppressive regimes and, therefore, in the account that follows, figures will frequently be given both for graft recipients with conventional immunosuppression and those receiving cyclosporin A. Immunosuppression with cyclosporin A has increased graft survival at one year[10] by about 12% (Figure 3.2). However, recent work by Dr D. B. Evans presented in a paper given at the Sandimmun Workshop, May 1988, has shown that the advantageous effect of cyclosporin A appears to be short term. In a 10-year study of 467 cadaveric renal transplants, he found that the graft survival after 6 years was superior in patients with azathioprine and prednisolone immunosuppression. The pattern of the survival curves of grafts with and without cyclosporin was different. Those with azathioprine and prednisolone had very few failures between 2 and 10 years, while those with cyclosporin had an inexorable graft loss of 5–6% per year. This preamble is required as considerable discussion has taken place recently concerning whether, in the age of cyclosporin A immunosuppression, HLA matching is still relevant to kidney graft survival, and, therefore, to the policy decision of whether it is desirable to transport cadaver kidneys from one transplant centre to another in order to graft them into the most compatible recipient.

It is necessary to consider kidney graft survival from living related and from cadaver donors separately. With living related donors, it is possible to identify whole haplotypes in common between donor and

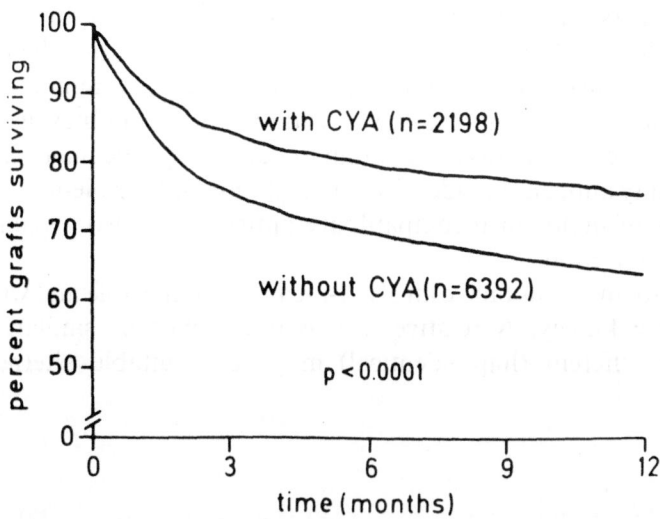

FIGURE 3.2   Survival of first cadaver kidney transplants in patients with or without cyclosporin treatment. Graft survival was computed by actuarial methods. The log rank test was used for calculation of statistical significance. Reproduced by permission from Opelz, G. (1985). Correlation of HLA matching with kidney graft survival in patients with or without cyclosporin treatment. *Transplantation*, **40**, 240–243 © by Williams & Wilkins

recipient, not just the antigens that we can currently demonstrate which act as markers for the haplotypes. If there is a haplotype identified in the recipient and in his family donor, this entails identity of at least one HLA-A, B, CW, DR, DP and DQ antigen.

GRAFT FROM A LIVING RELATED DONOR

An ABO-compatible HLA-identical sibling is the donor of choice for any patient needing a kidney transplant (Figure 3.3) The UCLA data on 1514 such transplants carried out since 1978 gives characteristic figures[11] with 77.8% of HLA-identical sibling kidney grafts func-

67

tioning 5 years after transplant. The amount of immunosuppression necessary for HLA-identical sibling grafts is minimal and therefore adverse side-effects of immunosuppression are also minimal. If, however, all immunosuppression is withdrawn, the kidney usually undergoes a rejection crisis, indicating that, although the major histocompatibility antigens are identical in the donor and recipient, incompatibilities of minor histocompatibility antigens are also capable of provoking rejection.

Most patients do not have an HLA-identical sibling able and willing to donate a kidney. A relative who is one haplotype similar, one haplotype different (haploidentical) may be a suitable alternative

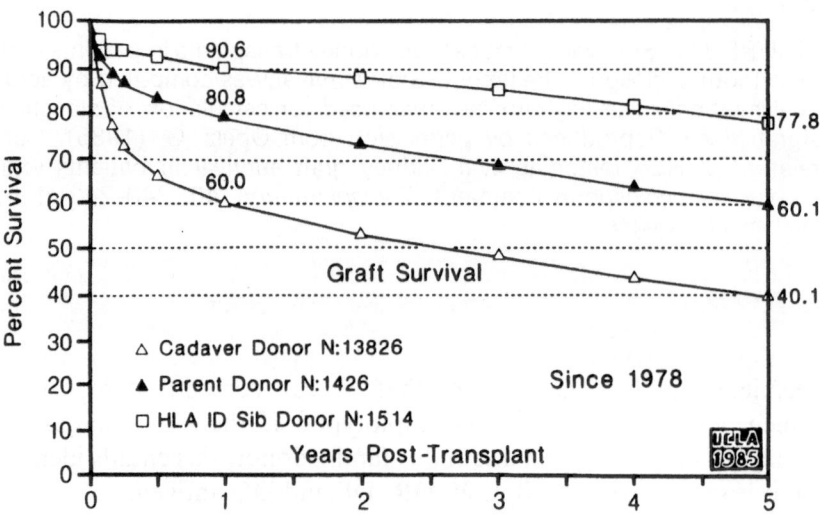

FIGURE 3.3   Five-year graft survival rates of first transplants performed after 1978. Of the transplants done since 1978, the 5-year graft survival was 77.8% for HLA-identical siblings, 60.1% for parental donors, and 40.1% for cadaver donors. It should be noted that there was a steady loss of transplants in all categories throughout the years. This applied even to HLA-identical siblings completely matched at the HLA locus[11]. By kind permission of Professor Terasaki and the publishers of *Clinical Kidney Transplants*, 1985

68

donor. Each parent transmits one haplotype to his or her offspring and therefore children automatically share one haplotype with each parent. They may also share one haplotype with a sibling, cousin or more distant relative. The survival of kidneys from a donor who is one haplotype similar, one haplotype different (haploidentical) e.g. a parent, is less good than that from an HLA-identical sibling donor (Figure 3.3). With a one-haplotype similar donor, there are incompatible antigens in the donor coded by the dissimilar haplotype that are not present in the recipient and these may provoke rejection. However, pretreatment of the recipient by blood transfusions from the donor (donor-specific transfusion, DST) in many cases greatly improves graft survival from a haploidentical donor[12]. On the other hand, DST may sensitize the patient to potential donor antigens and thereby render the recipient untransplantable from that donor. Recent multicentre studies have shown that, even when DST is employed, the survival of grafts is still lower than that for HLA identical grafts (Professor Opelz, Collaborative Transplant Study newsletter, May 1988).

GRAFT FROM AN UNRELATED CADAVER DONOR

Overall survival of cadaver donor kidney transplants is significantly less good than that of related grafts sharing one or two haplotypes (Figure 3.3)[11]. A cadaver donor is now routinely HLA typed for HLA-A, B and DR but, at present, partly because of the difficulty in obtaining good reagents, many laboratories do not usually type for HLA-CW, DP and DQ. In the family situation, if one or more haplotypes have been identified in common between donor and recipient, we can infer that other antigens coded by the haplotype bearing the HLA-A, B and DR antigens are also the same. We cannot necessarily make this inference with an unrelated donor. We have to define the difference between the donor and recipient by compatible and incompatible antigens rather than by haplotypes. An incompatible antigen is an antigen demonstrable in the donor that is not present in the recipient.

It is difficult to assess the effect of incompatibility of HLA antigens of a given locus in isolation, because the close linkage of the different

HLA loci often results in whole groups of antigens being incompatible rather than a single antigen. The polymorphism of the HLA antigens is sufficiently large that unless the transplant team actively select for similar antigens in donor and recipient, identity of HLA antigens, even at one locus, will rarely occur. For this reason, with random grafting it is very difficult to establish any effect of HLA matching as there are insufficient excellent matches for comparison.

The evaluation of the relevance of irrelevance of compatibility of donor/recipient tissue type on the survival of a kidney graft is fraught with pitfalls. The following are necessary for valid assessment of the effects of compatibility on graft survival: (1) good tissue typing, (2) numbers large enough to enable statistical significance to be obtained, (3) a follow-up period sufficiently long after transplantation to allow for long-term effects of incompatibility to show, and the time after transplant must be stated. For example, the statement that kidney grafts in a group had 95% survival is meaningless unless the time after transplant is stated and there should be contained in the material both 'excellent matches' and 'poor matches' for comparison.

HLA-A and B matching first grafts

When considering antigens controlled at any one locus, the maximum number of incompatibilities is 2 and therefore 4 incompatibilities at HLA-A and B represent a complete mismatch. In the literature, some authors describe the data in terms of antigen identities, while others describe comparable data in terms of incompatibilities or mismatches. Studies of the association between HLA compatibility and graft survival have had a chequered history, some teams reporting an association and some being unable to find any relationship. The large number of transplants recorded by collaborative studies have clarified the issue. The London Hospital Transplant Group[13] reported survival figures on 1340 transplants carried out before cyclosporin A was used. They found a statistically significant association ($p < 0.0001$) between compatibility of HLA-A and B and graft survival, such that there was a difference of 26% survival at 10 years between the best (41%) and the worst (15%) categories for HLA-A and B compatibility, i.e. HLA-A and B compatibility appeared to be relevant to long-term graft survival with conventional immunosuppression. Similarly, Cecka reported on 9499 conventionally immunosuppressed patients and found a 5-year survival of 50% if no HLA-A and B incompatibilities were present and 33% if there were four HLA-A and B incompatibilities, i.e. a 17% difference[14]. In patients receiving a cadaver graft immunosuppressed with cyclosporin A the effect of HLA-A and B matching at one year was present but was less than the effect with conventional immunosuppression. Persijn and colleagues found no clearcut statistically significant effect of HLA-A and B compatibility on graft survival at 1 and 2 years post-transplant on either conventionally immunosuppressed patients (2626 transplants) or those immunosuppressed with cyclosporin A (2909 transplants)[15]. Opelz[10] reported a statistically significant effect of HLA-A and B compatibility at one year on graft survival in those patients receiving conventional immunosuppression (6392 patients $p < 0.01$) and also those receiving cyclosporin A (2198 patients $p < 0.02$) (Figure 3.4)[10]. Although the ranking with the cyclosporin A patients was not strict, in both groups the difference between the percentage survival of the best and worst matches was about 10%. In summary, HLA-A and B compatibility was correlated with graft survival in the 5- and 10-year studies but in only some of the studies reported 1 and 2 years post-transplant.

Various authors have sought and not found a statistically significant effect of HLA-CW matching on graft survival[14]. However, Chapman and colleagues[16] reported hyperacute rejection attributable to anti-Cw5 present in a patient who received a kidney bearing Cw5.

HLA-DR antigen matching first grafts

Festenstein[13], Cecka[14], Persijn[15] and Opelz[10] and their collaborators in multicentre studies have demonstrated a statistically significant improvement in kidney graft survival with HLA-DR matching. In the Collaborative Transplant Study, with conventional immunosuppression, the effect of the HLA-DR matching graft survival at 1 year is statistically highly significant ($p < 0.0001$), the difference between the 'best' (no DR incompatibilities) and the 'worst' (two DR incompatibilities) being about 10% (Figure 3.5)[10]. Likewise, in the

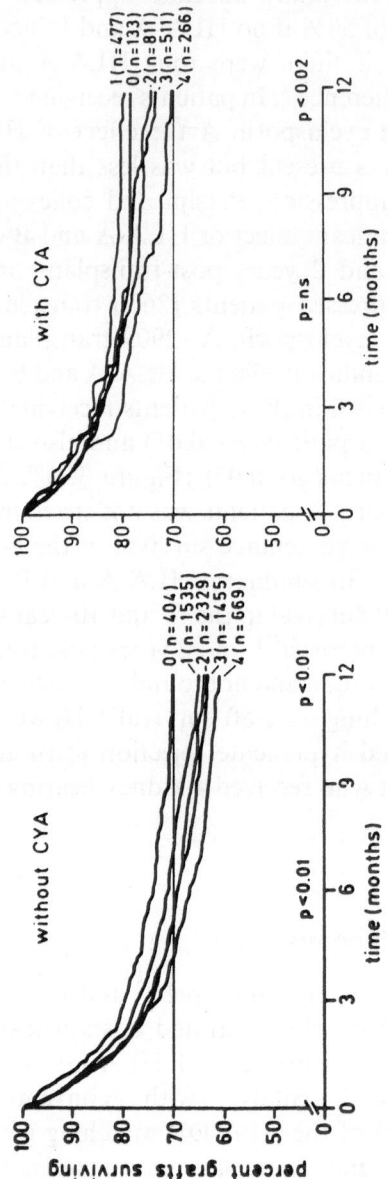

FIGURE 3.4   Analysis of HLA-A, B matching in first cadaver kidney transplants with or without cyclosporin treatment. Numbers of mismatched antigens are indicated at the end of curves and numbers of patients are given in parenthesis. Statistical significance was calculated by weighted regression analysis. The horizontal line at 70% was drawn to allow better comparison of the left half of the figure with the right half. Reproduced by permission from Opelz, G. (1985). Correlation of HLA matching with kidney graft survival in patients with or without cyclosporin treatment. *Transplantation*, **40**, 240–243 © by Williams & Wilkins

presence of cyclosporin A, the advantageous effect of matching for DR is about 10% and highly significant ($p < 0.001$). In contrast, an earlier multicentre study in 1983 of 232 patients in 8 centres (117 with cyclosporin A and 115 with conventional immunosuppression) failed to find evidence of benefit of HLA-A, B or DR matching at one-year follow-up[17].

Madsen and colleagues[18] in a study 6 months post-transplant were able to demonstrate improved graft survival associated with DR compatibility when azathioprine immunosuppression was used, but the effect was not demonstrable in 71 patients treated with cyclosporin A. However, the authors comment that only one patient in the cyclosporin A group was poorly matched, i.e. had two DR incompatibilities, so, for comparative purposes, the series was not satisfactory.

Using a functional assessment of graft survival, instead of death of the kidney, a study[19] of 84 cadaver transplants from one centre using cyclosporin A examined the effect of DR incompatibilities on the following factors: (1) plasma creatinine levels, (2) necessity for investigative biopsy, (3) histological assessment of rejection, (4) length of time in hospital, (5) crude graft survival. Failure of the grafted kidney was not significantly associated with DR incompatibility, but transplants with zero DR incompatibilities compared with those possessing 1 or 2 incompatibilities showed significantly lower plasma creatinine levels at 1-year post-transplant, needed significantly fewer investigative biopsies, showed significantly fewer examples of histologically defined rejection, and also needed shorter periods of hospitalization. The last factor can, of course, be influenced by a large number of factors, but rapid discharge from hospital with a functioning kidney does not usually occur if the patient is rejecting!

Combined effect of compatibility of HLA-B and HLA-DR of first grafts

When the transplant data were analysed in relation to combined incompatibilities at HLA-DR and HLA-B, highly significant correlations with graft survival have been found by Festenstein et al.[13], Cecka[14] and Opelz[10]. The last two authors showed that the improvement occurs both with conventional immunosuppression and with

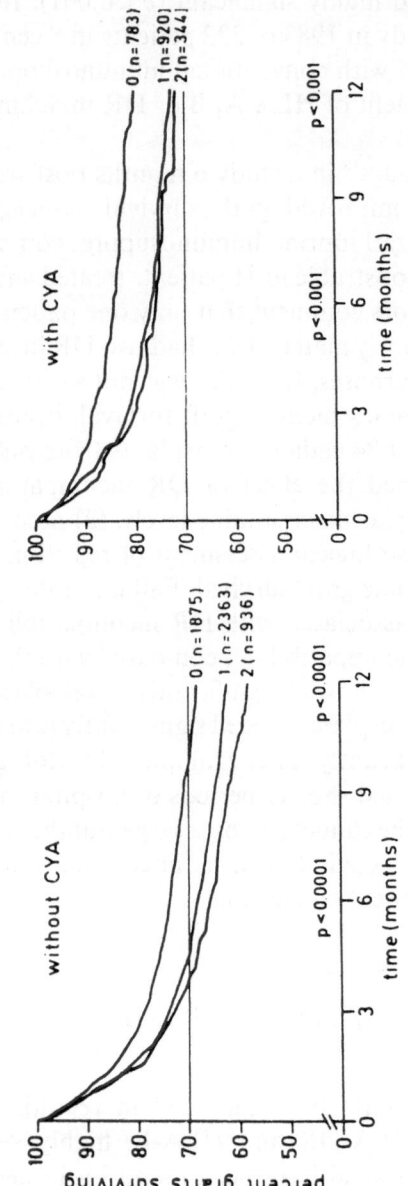

FIGURE 3.5   Effect of HLA-DR matching on first cadaver kidney transplants. Success rates were higher for grafts with no HLA-DR mismatches, with or without cyclosporin treatment. Statistical significance at 6 and 12 months was determined by weighted regression. Reproduced by permission from Opelz, G. (1985). Correlation of HLA matching with kidney graft survival in patients with or without cyclosporin treatment. *Transplantation*, **40**, 240–243 © by Williams & Wilkins

cyclosporin A. Figure 3.6, from Opelz[10], shows a stepwise effect of the compatibility of the HLA-B and HLA-DR antigens on graft survival, such that the difference between the best (0 incompatibilities at HLA-B and DR) and the worst matches (4 incompatibilities) was about 20% at 1 year. The effect was present both with conventional immunosuppression and with cyclosporin A. The improvements in graft survival attributable to cyclosporin A and HLA-B and DR matching were additive.

Gilks and colleagues[20] carried out a rigorous statistical analysis of the combined effects of HLA-A, B and DR matching in 2282 first cadaver kidney transplants contributed to the United Kingdom Transplant Service (UKTS). They compared survival of the transplants one year after grafting according to the number (0, 1 or 2) of incompatibilities at the HLA-A, B and DR loci. They did not differentiate for type of immunosuppressive therapy. They found that there was substantial benefit to the recipient if there were zero incompatibilities at DR, and a maximum of 1 incompatibility at either HLA-A *or* HLA-B (Table 3.3). They designated the top three categories 'beneficially matched' and indicated that, in their study, they could demonstrate little advantage if lesser degrees of HLA matching were present.

Opelz (1988)[21] has recently examined graft survival in relation to HLA compatibility assessed in two ways. HLA-A and B antigens can be defined either as broad specificities, e.g. HLA-A9, or as narrow subspecificities or splits, e.g. HLA-A23 or A24 (Table 3.1). Correlation between HLA matching and graft survival was very much stronger if subspecificities rather than specificities were used to define HLA-A and B antigens, both when they were considered alone and in combination with HLA-DR. For HLA-A and B matching, when broad antigens were considered, there was no obvious correlation with graft survival, but, when antigen splits were taken into account, the difference between survival of grafts with 0 and 4 mismatches was 18% at 3 years (p log rank < 0.0001). Similarly when HLA-DR and HLA-A and B subspecificities were considered together, there was a 31% difference in survival between grafts with 0 and 6 mismatches at 3 years (Figure 3.7; p log rank < 0.0001). This effect was present both in the presence of conventional immunosuppression and cyclosporin A. This suggests that the early inconclusive results of the effect of

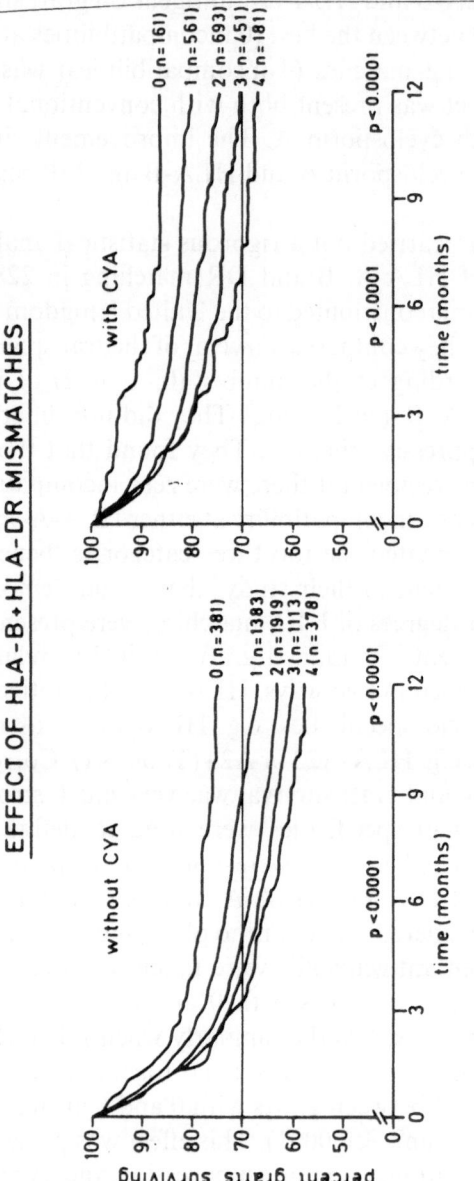

FIGURE 3.6 Combined analysis of HLA-B and HLA-DR matching in first cadaver kidney transplants. Number of mismatched antigens is indicated for each subgroup at the end of the curve. number of patients studied is given in parenthesis. There was a progressive decline in graft survival from 0 to 4 mismatches, with or without cyclosporin. Statistical significance was calculated by weighted regression analysis. Reproduced by permission from Opelz, G. (1985). Correlation of HLA matching with kidney graft survival in patients with or without cyclosporin treatment. *Transplantation*, **40**, 240–243 © by Williams & Wilkins

TABLE 3.3   Graft survival and HLA matching in first cadaver kidney transplants, UKTS data

HLA-(A, B, DR) mismatches	% 1-year graft survival	Number of grafts	Defined according to reference 20
0, 0, 0	93	73	} 'beneficially matched'
1, 0, 0	86	108	
0, 1, 0	81	97	
0, 0, 1	67	96	} 'not beneficially matched'
2 in total	73	603	
3 in total	70	720	
4 in total	71	399	
5 in total	65	154	

Based on data from Gilks and colleagues[20]. The data were estimated multifactorially, controlling for transplant centre and year of transplant

HLA matching on graft survival may have been partly attributable to too wide a definition of the HLA-A and B antigens.

A sensitized patient, who has anti-HLA antibody reacting against a large proportion of the population, may have to wait a very long time before a crossmatch-negative donor becomes available. In addition, graft survival in highly sensitized patients is significantly less good ($p < 0.001$) than in unsensitized or weakly sensitized patients (Figure 3.8)[22]. The difference in survival of grafts between those patients who are unsensitized and those who are sensitized to more than 50% of the population is not reduced by cyclosporin A[22] (Figure 3.8).

We have seen in the unsensitized patients that the effect of HLA-A and B matching on graft survival was demonstrable in some studies but not in others and in the Collaborative Transplant Study was about 10% one year post-transplant. In those patients who had antibody in their latest (current) serum sample against more than 50% of the population, the effect of HLA-A and B matching was increased and became highly significant ($p < 0.001$) such that grafts with zero HLA-A and B mismatches had a graft survival at one year of more

WITH CYCLOSPORIN
ANTIGEN SPLITS

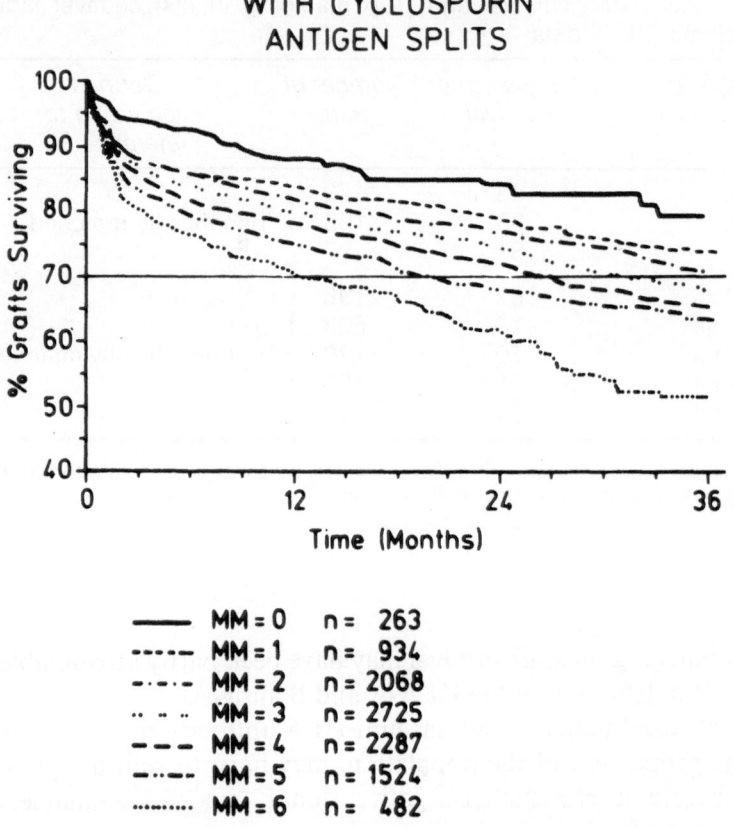

—— MM = 0	n =	263
-----· MM = 1	n =	934
-·-·- MM = 2	n =	2068
·· - ·· MM = 3	n =	2725
— — — MM = 4	n =	2287
—··—· MM = 5	n =	1524
·········· MM = 6	n =	482

FIGURE 3.7   Effect of mismatching for antigen splits of HLA-A and B together with DR on first kidneys in cyclosporin-treated patients[21]. By kind permission of Professor Opelz and the publishers of *The Lancet*

than 15% above those with a complete HLA-A and B mismatch[22] (Figure 3.9).

In unsensitized patients, the combined effect of HLA-B and DR matching has been shown to be significant and additive and gives an improvement in graft survival of about 20% at one year. In patients with antibodies reacting with more than 50% of the population, the advantageous effect of combined HLA-B and DR matching is increased and is highly significant ($p < 0.0001$); with both conventional immunosuppression and with cyclosporin A, the advantageous

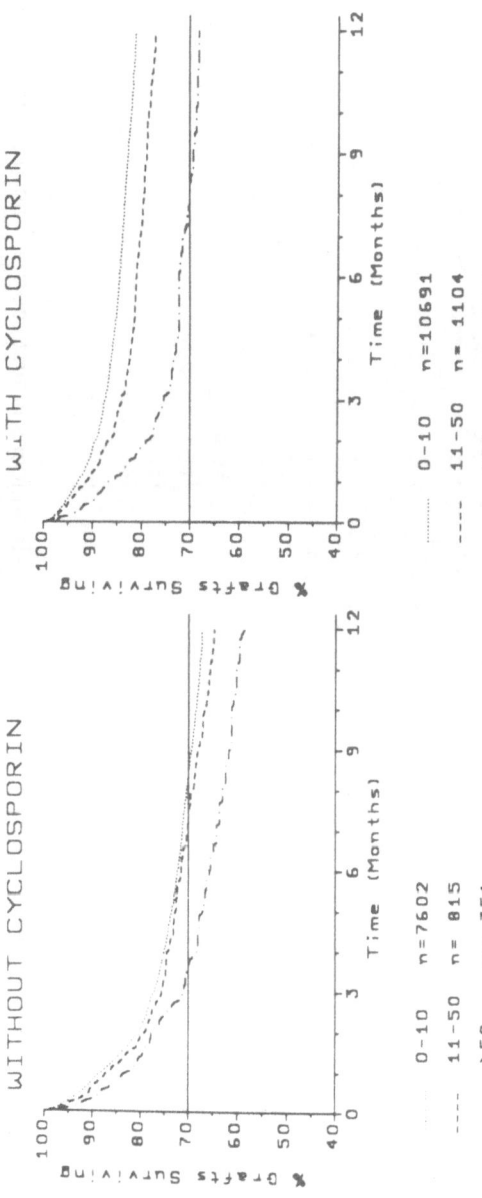

FIGURE 3.8   Influence of preformed lymphocytotoxic antibodies on graft survival in patients treated with or without cyclosporin. Percentage of antibody reactivity against panel and number of patients studied is indicated for each curve[22]. By kind permission of Professor Opelz and the publishers of *Transplantation Proceedings*

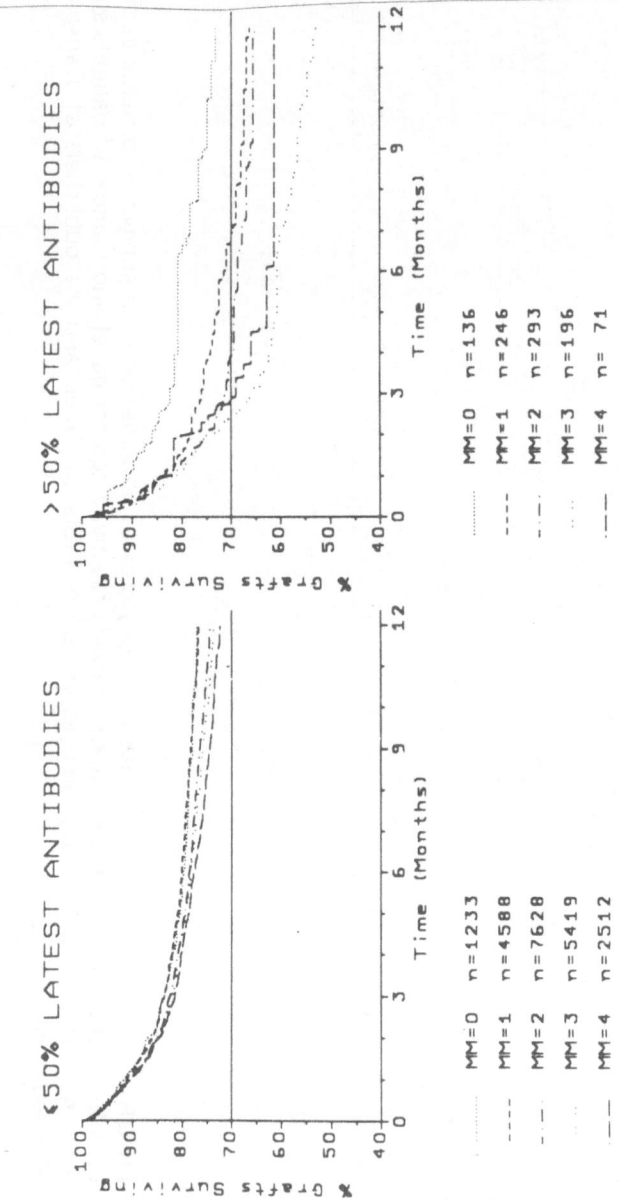

FIGURE 3.9 Effect of matching for HLA-A and HLA-B antigens in first cadaver transplant recipients with <50% (p<0.0001) or ≥50% (p <0.001) preformed lymphocytotoxic antibodies[22]. By kind permission of Professor Opelz and the publishers of *Transplantation Proceedings*

increment was between 25 and 30%[22] (Figure 3.10). In other words, in sensitized patients who have antibodies against more than 50% of the population, matching for HLA-B and HLA-DR can improve graft survival at one year by between 25 and 30%. We now await with interest information on the relevance of matching for antigen splits on the graft survival in sensitized patients.

Cadaver grafts – survival of first, second and subsequent grafts

Overall survival of first grafts tends to be superior to that of second grafts[23].

Even in the presence of immunosuppression, incompatible HLA antigens in a rejected transplant frequently provoke the production of cytotoxic antibody. In a sample of patients who had rejected their grafted kidney, Sanfillipo and colleagues[24] showed that there was a significant association between the degree of HLA-A and B incompatibility in the first graft and the development of cytotoxic antibody, such that poorly matched grafts provoked cytotoxic antibody against a larger proportion of the population than did well-matched grafts. Presence of cytotoxic antibody against a large proportion of the population limits the choice of possible donors and a sensitized patient may have to wait a long time before a kidney can be found that gives a negative crossmatch.

The advantageous effect of HLA-DR and B matching on second grafts is very similar to that of patients who have more than 50% cytotoxic antibody, namely the difference in survival between donor/recipient HLA-B and DR identity and complete disparity is more than 20% at one year post-transplant[22] (Figure 3.11).

Anomalies in the correlation between HLA matching and graft survival

Some allografts are poorly matched and function satisfactorily for a prolonged period of time while others appear to be well matched and fail. It follows that factors other than simple compatibility of HLA as presently defined are also of importance in allograft survival. All antigens even at one locus are not equal in effect. Hendriks and colleagues[25] reported that DRw6 recipients appear to be 'high respon-

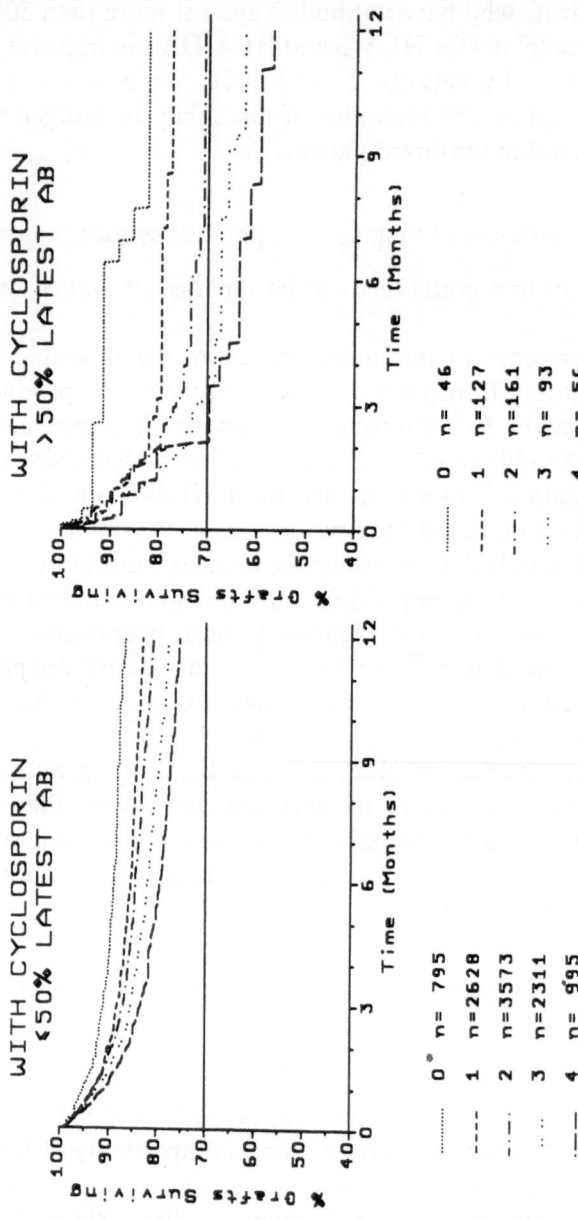

FIGURE 3.10 Effect of matching for HLA-B and HLA-DR antigens in cyclosporin-treated recipients of first cadavar transplants. The matching effect is stronger in patients with >50% antibody reactivity (p <0.0001) than in patients with ≤50% reactivity (p <0.001). The latest pretransplant serum was analysed[22]. By kind permission of Professor Opelz and the publishers of *Transplantation Proceedings*

82

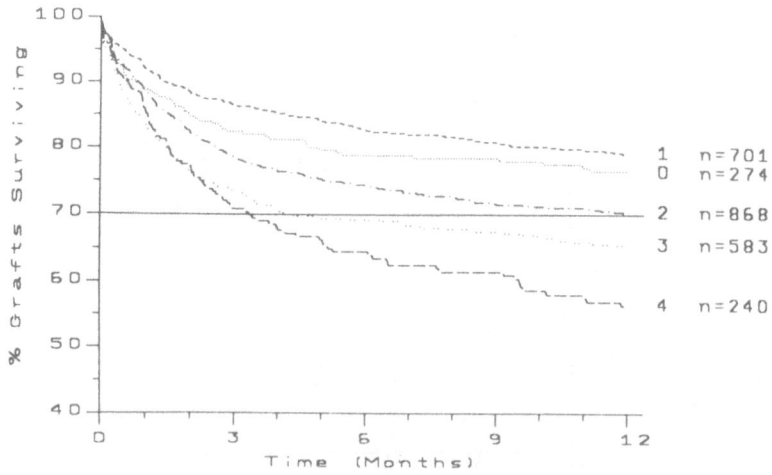

FIGURE 3.11 Effect of mismatches for HLA-B and HLA-DR on outcome of second cadaver kidney transplants. All patients were immunosuppressed with cyclosporin. The number of mismatches antigens and numbers of patients studied are indicated[31]. By kind permission of Professor Opelz and the publishers of *Transplantation Proceedings*

ders' to foreign DR antigen (i.e. respond very vigorously) so that the differences between graft survival of the best and worst DR matches are considerably greater in patients with DRw6 than in those lacking this antigen (Figures 3.12a and b)[25]. In addition, DRw6 in the donor was reported to have an unexplained advantageous effect on graft survival whether or not the antigen is compatible[26]. These effects of DRw6 were confirmed by Vereerstraetan and colleagues[27]. In contrast to the DRw6 recipient effect, Cook[28] has shown that patients bearing DR1 are 'lower responders' to foreign DR antigens and have an overall graft survival superior to that of recipients of other groups.

Policies employed in UK in relation to tissue typing and kidney transplantation

There is no one policy that is adhered to by all transplant centres. Most centres do not knowingly graft ABO incompatible kidneys, and

83

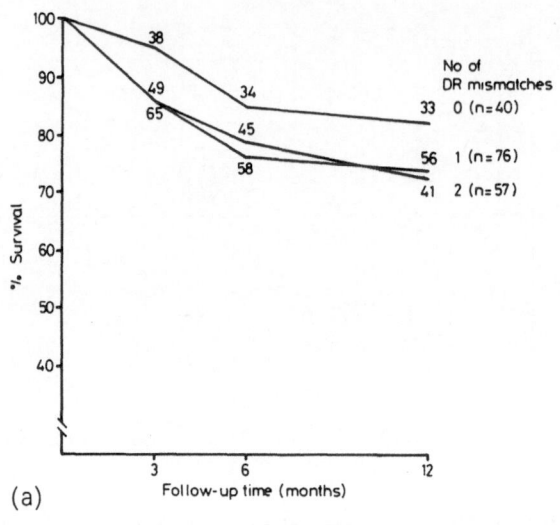

(a)

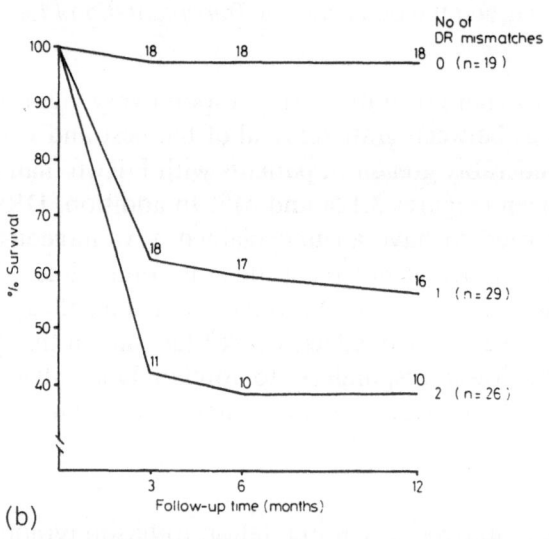

(b)

FIGURE 3.12   To show the effect of HLA-DR mismatches on survival of first grafts in (a) 173 recipients who are HLA-DRw6 negative in comparison with (b) 74 recipients who are DRw6 positive[25]. By kind permission of Dr Hendriks and the publishers of *British Medical Journal*

most carry out a lymphocytotoxic crossmatch of the serum of the recipient on the lymphocytes of the donor prior to transplant. If the immediate pretransplant serum sample gives a positive crossmatch due to an IgG anti-HLA antibody, the transplant is not usually carried out as hyperacute rejection is likely to supervene. Centres differ in the importance that they ascribe to a 'historical' crossmatch. Some centres will graft if the crossmatch with a historical serum sample is positive as long as the crossmatch with the immediate pretransplant serum sample is negative.

Policy of different centres is also diverse in relation to the weight that is given to HLA matching. Some centres do not attempt to HLA match but graft a kidney into a recipient using only the criteria of ABO compatibility, crossmatch negativity and clinical urgency. Most British centres and many elsewhere now use the majority of kidneys harvested in their local area on their own recipients using ABO and negative crossmatch criteria and attempting to get the best HLA match possible on their local recipients; they rarely give kidneys to the national pool unless they have no ABO-compatible crossmatch-negative recipients. This policy has increased since the use of cyclosporin A in the mistaken impression that cyclosporin A ablates the effect of HLA matching. This can result in a patient receiving a kidney mismatched on all detectable HLA antigens and often results in a rejected kidney and a highly sensitized patient.

Some centres utilize kidneys harvested from a donor by grafting one kidney into the best matched local recipient and giving the other to the national pool for the most beneficially matched recipient in the country.

The cytomegalovirus (CMV) status of the kidney donor and recipient can complicate an HLA matching policy; after transplant, an immunosuppressed patient may develop a CMV infection which is usually derived either from a CMV-positive donor or by reactivation of a previous infection in the recipient[29,30]. The clinically most severe infections, which may be lethal, tend to be in CMV-seronegative patients who have received a CMV-positive kidney[29]. For this reason, some centres now attempt to 'match' donor and recipient for CMV status so that a CMV antibody-negative donor is considered for all potential recipients but a CMV-positive donor is considered only for CMV-positive recipients. This may reduce the number of deaths from

CMV disease but it also reduces the possible pool of donors available for the CMV-negative patient. If this policy is pursued, they can be expected to have to wait longer than the CMV-positive individual for a good match. Smiley and colleagues[29] suggest vaccination against CMV to seroconvert their patients and observe that reactivation after transplant does not seem to occur in patients so treated.

Organ sharing schemes

The foregoing account illustrates that HLA matching of kidney donor and recipient can confer substantial benefit to the recipient of a first graft and the effect is greater for sensitized patients and for recipients of second and subsequent grafts. Collaborative organ sharing schemes are in operation in many countries to exchange kidneys between transplant centres on the basis of good HLA matching, e.g. UK Transplant Service. The facilities of organ exchange are greatly under-used.

Four reasons are often given by transplant centres for non-collaboration in organ-sharing programmes:

(1) Some centres are unable to demonstrate correlation between HLA matching and graft survival in their own single-centre series and therefore they distrust the data from thousands of transplants with follow-up of many years. This is a scientifically suspect view, as, however good the transplant centre, unless it is using fundamentally different immunosuppression from that in other centres, the biological rules governing rejection worked out on collaborative data are likely to hold true.

(2) Centres may distrust results of DR typing at their own and other centres on which organ exchange is partly based. At present, results of DR typing are not perfect but they are rapidly improving. However, it should be remembered that the collaborative transplant studies in which large significant effects of DR typing were demonstrated were carried out with current methods. If, in the presence of admitted inaccuracy, these results were obtained, the effects of matching must be very strong.

(3) Tissue typing, computer matching and transport of kidneys may take many hours and it has been argued that, especially with the use of cyclosporin A, the acceptable ischaemia time would be exceeded. However, in a series of 14 065 transplants treated with cyclosporin A, with a range of ischaemia times, Opelz found that no significant decrease in graft survival up to 1 year was demonstrable until the ischaemia time exceeded 48 hours[31].

(4) Surgical teams put an enormous amount of effort into harvesting kidneys and they may fear that they will 'lose' them to other centres who may be less active or less skilled in kidney procurement. This may happen, but a system of 'fair shares' has been proposed by United Kingdom Transplant Service that, in the event of two equally matched recipients being from different centres, the recipient from the centre that has put the larger proportion of kidneys into the pool would 'win' the kidney.

Success?

Central to the definition of a policy that would be optimal for the patient is the question: what are the criteria of success? A patient's criterion of complete success would probably be to have no rejection episodes, to leave hospital within two weeks of transplant and to achieve a kidney functioning within the normal range for the rest of his or her natural lifespan.

What actually happens?

Cyclosporin A improves graft survival by about 12% at 1 year. In addition to this, when combined HLA-DR and B matching is optimal, the clear results of multicentre studies show improvement is graft survival of up to 20% at 1 year for first grafts, and, with highly sensitized and retransplant patients, the improvement at 1 year may be about 30%. If it is possible to achieve a good match, a policy decision to ignore HLA matching represents a failure to take steps to prevent 10–30% of the patients from returning to dialysis after 1 year, probably sensitized. However, in many cases, despite indifferent matching, the grafted kidney will function for several years before the patient returns to dialysis.

A dilemma faces transplant units: they have a large number of patients on dialysis awaiting transplant and a totally inadequate number of kidneys to supply the need. At the time of writing, in the UK there are 2828 people on the list awaiting a transplant but, in 1987, only 1562 kidneys were available. There is pressure on dialysis slots and some of the patients are clinically urgent. In this context, it is not surprising that when a surgical team harvests kidneys they usually use them on patients in their own centre. Even in centres that aim to achieve HLA matching, the polymorphism of HLA renders it unlikely that optimal matching will be achieved very often when a small number of local donors is available.

Although it may be desirable, is a well-matched kidney a logistically achievable aim for a given patient? The answer to this question depends on several factors. The first and most important factor is the size of

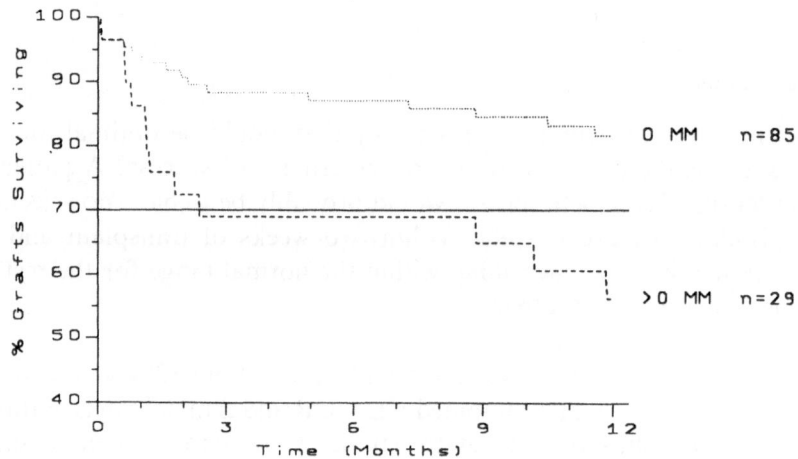

FIGURE 3.13   Graft survival analysis of cadaver donor kidneys of HLA type A1, B8 and DR3. No other HLA antigens were found in the donors. Because families of cadaver donors usually are not HLA typed, these kidneys were considered operationally homozygous for the purpose of kidney sharing. The 85 transplants without mismatch between donor and recipient survived at a significantly higher rate than the 29 transplants that were mismatched ($p < 0.01$)[31]. By kind permission of Professor Opelz and the publishers of *Transplantation Proceedings*

the donor pool from which a kidney can be drawn. It follows that, if all kidneys were given to the national pool, then the chance of a patient receiving a well-matched graft would be much greater than if only local donors could be drawn on. Gilks et al.[20] calculated that, at present in the UK, only 12.5% of grafts are 'beneficially matched', i.e. on their definition, there are no incompatibilities on DR and a maximum of one on HLA-A and B. However, computer simulation studies from the United Kingdom Transplant Service indicate that, with a recipient list of 3000 and 3000 donor kidneys, if the kidneys were given to the best-matched recipient in the UK, 60% of patients awaiting transplant could receive a 'beneficially matched' kidney (Table 3.3).

The second factor is the tissue type of the recipient. Some haplotypes are common, e.g. A1, B8, DR3. Opelz[31] reported that, among 29 771 transplant recipients reported to the Collaborative Transplant Study, 3506 (i.e. 11.8%) possessed this antigen combination, although most had other antigens as well. In the same series of transplants, 114 cadaver kidneys available for transplant had no other demonstrable HLA antigens, i.e. the donors appeared to be homozygous. It would have been possible for every one of these kidneys to have been transplanted into a recipient with zero HLA-A, B or DR incompatibilities but this happened for only 85/114 patients; 12 kidneys were transplanted into recipients with 1 incompatibility, 9 with 2 incompatibilities and 8 with 3 incompatibilities. In this small but antigenically homogeneous group, the survival at one year was more than 20% better in the 'matched' than in the 'mismatched' group (Figure 3.13)[31]. The kidneys that were 'used up' locally on poorly matched recipients could almost certainly have given better service to recipients with no HLA incompatibilities at other centres. More than 40% of the recipients that received poorly matched grafts after one year had lost their kidney and some/most would have to be returned to the recipient list for a second transplant. It would have been perfectly possible and better to get it right the first time!

For the patient with rarer groups, it may be genuinely difficult to obtain a good match, but, even here, it should be possible to obtain HLA-DR compatibility. Likewise, the clinically urgent patient may not be able to wait for an optimal HLA match, but, if all donor kidneys were exchanged, most should be able to get a reasonably well-

89

matched kidney. The policy that is at present exercised by many centres, of using nearly all donor kidneys on the nearest HLA matched recipient in the centre that harvested the kidneys, gives reasonably good short-term results judged by crude graft survival thanks to cyclosporin A. The number of well-matched grafts achieved and therefore the long-term survival are both less than they could be.

Kidneys are in short supply but those that are available for transplant are not being used to the greatest efficiency. Many that might have been put into a well-matched recipient and given many years of service are instead rejected by a poorly matched recipient. This is a waste and in many cases is avoidable. The best use of the precious resource of available cadaver kidneys is that each kidney should be transplanted into the recipient in whom it is most likely to succeed. This can best be achieved if the kidneys are exchanged between centres on the basis of advantageous HLA matching.

If the majority of transplanted kidneys were good matches, this would result in better long-term survival than at present and consequently fewer second and subsequent transplants would be needed. This, in itself, would reduce the need for kidneys, the necessity for expensive investigative biopsy, antirejection therapy and long-term hospitalization would be less. In this instance, for once, national economics and humanity point in the same direction, towards donation of all available kidneys to the most advantageously matched recipient. This will only be achieved, however, by consensus of the transplant teams. United Kingdom Transplant Service has circulated (July 1988) the head of each transplant unit in the UK requesting collaboration in a scheme in which UKTS be informed of the tissue type of every kidney donor as soon as the information becomes available, and, if there is a beneficially matched recipient in the country, that the kidney be given to that patient. If all transplant units participate in this collaboration, computer simulation studies[20] indicate that 60% of kidney recipients would receive 'beneficially matched' kidneys. If there was no 'beneficially matched' potential recipient available, as would happen 40% of the time, then the kidney(s) would be retained by the procuring transplant centre for use on their own recipients, as happens at present. If this plan is accepted by the transplant centres, then donor kidneys will be used to the best advantage of all patients.

90

Acknowledgements

The author would like to thank Mrs A. Cowell for excellent secretarial help.

REFERENCES

1. Counce, S., Smith, P., Barth, R. and Snell, G. D. (1956) Strong and weak histocompatibility gene differences in mice and their role in the rejection of homografts of tumours and skin. *Ann. Surg.*, **144**, 198–204
2. Breimer, M. W., Brynger, H., Le Pendu, J., Oriol, R., Rydberg, L., Samuelsson, B. E. and Vinas, J. (1987). Blood group ABO-incompatible kidney transplantation biochemical and immunochemical studies of blood group A glycolipid antigens in human kidney and characterization of the antibody response (antigen specificity and antibody class) in 0 recipients receiving A₂ grafts. *Transplant. Proc.*, **19**, 226–230
3. Rydberg, L., Breimer, M. E., Samuelsson, B. E. and Brynger, H. (1987). Blood group ABO-incompatible (A₂ to 0) kidney transplantation in human subjects: a clinical, serologic, and biochemical aproach. *Transplant. Proc.*, **19**, 4528–4537
4. Welsh, K. I., van Dam, M., Koffman, C. G., Bewick, M. E., Rudge, C. J., Tuabe, D. H. and Clark, A. G. B. (1987). Transplantation of blood group A₂ kidneys into 0 or B recipients: the effect of pretransplant anti-A titers on graft survival. *Transplant. Proc.*, **19**, 4565–4567
5. Shapira, Z., Yussim, A., Shmueli, D. and Nakache, R. (1987). Experience with blood group A₂ renal grafts in ABO-incompatible recipients. *Transplant Proc.*, **19**, 4562–4564
6. Cook, D. J., Graver, B. and Terasaki, P. I. (1987). ABO incompatibility in cadaver donor kidney allografts. *Transplant Proc.*, **19**, 4549–4552
7. Ting, A. and Morris, P. J. (1983). Successful transplantation with a positive T and B cell crossmatch due to autoreactive antibodies. *Tissue Antigens*, **21**, 219–226
8. Falk, J. A., Cardella, C. J., Halloran, P., Robinette, M., Arbus, G. and Bear, R. (1985). Transplantation can be performed with positive (noncurrent) crossmatch. *Transplant. Proc.*, **17**, 1530–1532
9. Kerman, R. H., Flechner, S. M., Van Buren, C. T., Lorber, M. I. and Kahan, B. D. (1985). Successful transplantation of cyclosporine treated allograft recipients with serologically positive historical, but negative preoperative, donor crossmatches. *Transplantation*, **40**, 615–619
10. Opelz, G. (1985). Correlation of HLA matching with kidney graft survival in patients with or without cyclosporine treatment. *Transplantation*, **40**, 240–243
11. Terasaki, P. I., Toyotome, A., Mickey, M. R., Cicciarelli, J., Iwaki, Y., Cecka, M. and Tiwari, J. (1985). Patient, graft, and functional survival rates: an overview. In Terasali, P. I. (ed.) *Clinical Kidney Transplants*, Chapt. 1, pp. 1–26. (California: UCLA Tissue Typing Laboratory)
12. Salvatierra, O., Vicenti, F., Amend, W., Carovoy, M., Iwaki, Y., Terasaki, P., Potter, D., Duca, R., Hopper, S., Slemmer, T. and Feduska, N. (1983). Four-

year experience with donor-specific blood transfusion. *Transplant. Proc.*, **15**, 924–931

13. Festenstein. H., Doyle, P. and Holmes, J. (1986). Long-term follow-up in London Transplant Group recipients of cadaver renal allografts. *N. Engl. J. Med.*, **314**, 7–13

14. Cecka, J. M. (1986). The changing role of HLA matching. In Terasaki, P. I. (ed.) *Clinical Transplants*, Chapt. 16, pp. 141–155. (California: UCLA Tissue Typing Laboratory)

15. Persijn, G. G., de Lange, P., D'Amaro, J., Cohen, B., Liebelt, P., Hendriks, G. F. J. and van Rood, J. J. (1986). Eurotransplant Part II. The cyclosporine era 1981–1985. In Terasaki, P. I. (ed.) *Clinical Transplants*, Chapt. 13, pp. 99–107. (California: UCLA Tissue Typing Laboratory)

16. Chapman, J. R., Taylor, C., Ting, A. and Morris, P. J. (1986). Hyperacute rejection of a renal allograft in the presence of anti-CW5 antibody. *Transplantation*, **42**, No. 1, 91–92

17. European Multicentre Trial Group (1983). Cyclosporin in cadaveric renal transplantation: one-year follow-up of a multicentre trial. *Lancet*, **2**, 986–989

18. Madsen, M., Graugaard, B., Fjeldborg, O., Hansen, H. E., Posborg, V. and Kissmeyer-Nielsen (1985). The impact of HLA-DR antigen matching in cyclosporine-treated recipients of cadaveric renal allografts. A single-center analysis. *Transplant. Proc.*, **17**, No. 6, 2202–2204

19. Joysey, V. C., Thiru, S. and Evans, D. B. (1985). Effect of HLA-DR compatibility on kidney transplants treated with cyclosporine A. *Transplant. Proc.*, **17**, No. 6, 2187–2192

20. Gilks, W. R., Bradley, B. A., Gore, S. M. and Klouda, P. T. (1987). Substantial benefits of tissue matching in renal transplantation. *Transplantation*, **43**, No. 5, 669–673

21. Opelz, G. (1988). Importance of HLA antigen splits for kidney transplant matching. *Lancet*, **2**, 61–64

22. Opelz, G. (1987). Kidney transplantation in sensitized patients. *Transplant. Proc.*, **19**, No. 5, 3737–3741

23. Iwaki, Y. and Terasaki, P. I. (1986). Sensitization effect. In Terasaki, P. I. (ed.) *Clinical Transplants*, Chapt. 25, pp. 257–265. (California: UCLA Tissue Typing Laboratory)

24. Sanfilippo, F., Goeken, G., Niblack, G., Scornik, J. and Vaughn, W. K. (1987). The impact of HLA-A, B match of primary renal allografts subsequent to transplant failure. *Transplant. Proc.*, **19**, 669–671

25. Hendriks, G. F. J., Schreuder, G. M. Th., Claas, F. H. J., D'Amaro, J., Persijn, G. G., Cohen, B. and van Rood, J. J. (1983). HLA-DRw6 and renal allograft rejection. *Br. Med. J.*, **286**, 85–87

26. Hendriks, C. F. J., D'Amaro, J., Pensijn, G. G., Schreuder, G. M. T., Lansbergen, Q., Cohen, B. and van Rood, J. J. (1983). Excellent outcome after transplantation of renal allografts from HLA-DRw6 positive donors even in HLA-DR mismatches. *Lancet*, **2**, 187–189

27. Vereerstraeten, P., Andrien, M., Dupont, E., De Pauw, L., Kinnaert, P. and Toussaint, C. (1987). Influence of donor and recipient DRw6 status on outcome of cadaver kidney transplantation. *Transplant. Proc.*, **19**, No. 1, 708–710

28. Cook, D. J. (1986). HLA-DR associated immune responsiveness. In Terasaki, P. I. (ed.) *Clinical Transplants*, Chapt. 24, pp. 247–256. (California: UCLA Tissue Typing Laboratory)

29. Smiley, M. L., Wlodaver, C. G., Grossman, R. A., Barker, C. F., Perloff, L. J., Tustin, N. B., Starr, S. E., Plotkin, S. A. and Friedman, H. M. (1985). The role of pretransplant immunity in protection from cytomegalovirus disease following renal transplantation. *Transplantation*, **40**, No. 2, 157–161

30. Grundy, J. E., Lui, S. F., Super, M., Berry, N. J., Sweny, P., Fernando, O. N., Moorhead, J. and Griffiths, P. D. (1988). Symptomatic cytomegalovirus infection in seropositive kidney recipients: reinfection with donor virus rather than reactivation of recipient virus. *Lancet*, **2**, 132–135

31. Opelz, G. (1988). Allocation of cadaver kidneys for transplantation. *Transplant. Proc.*, **20**, No. 1, Suppl. 1, 1028–1032

4
IMMUNOLOGICAL MONITORING

A. I. LAZAROVITS and C. R. STILLER

INTRODUCTION

A successful renal transplant is the most desirable form of therapy for the management of end-stage renal disease in suitable patients. These people are offered an excellent opportunity to be rehabilitated and to lead a more normal lifestyle. Furthermore, a great deal of money is saved for the health care system[1]; and, for patients with end-stage disease of other organs, such as heart, liver and lungs, a successful transplant is virtually the only hope for survival.

While patient survival after renal transplantation is excellent[2] (less than 5% mortality per year), and while this compares very favourably with the survival statistics associated with the therapy of other diseases, the chances for a successful engraftment are not so good. The Canadian Multicentre Transplant Study Group has recently shown that patients who are treated with cyclosporin and prednisone have a 30% risk of losing their grafts at the end of three years, the vast majority from rejection[2].

Thus, rejection remains the single largest impediment to success in this field of transplantation. Part of the problem is our inability to make an early diagnosis of rejection before the usual clinical signs and symptoms appear. An early diagnosis would allow treatment to be started before damage to the allograft occurred. Furthermore, immunosuppressive therapy could be reduced if it were accurately known when rejection activity ceased; this would decrease the morbidity and even mortality associated with over-immunosuppression.

There is, therefore, a pressing need for the development of a sensitive and specific test which would allow one to differentiate between the various causes of renal allograft dysfunction. The hope would be to differentiate between rejection, infection, cyclosporin nephrotoxicity, and acute tubular necrosis, which are the major diagnostic dilemmas.

One approach to this problem is based upon recent advances in transplant immunology and our improved understanding of the intricate mechanisms that ultimately determine the success or failure of a transplant. This review will attempt to summarize a wide variety of recent advances in the field of immunological monitoring. Topics to be covered will be the evaluation of the patient both pre- and post-transplant, including HLA, the vascular endothelial cell monocyte system, red blood cells, the type and specificity of preformed antibodies and the proliferative capacity of the lymphocytes. Post-transplant topics will include core and fine-needle aspiration biopsies and a thorough characterization of the structure and function of the infiltrating cells. Other areas to be covered will be the evaluation of the recipient for immunologic responses to specific antigens of the graft donor, such as cell-mediated lymphocytotoxicity and complement-dependent antibody assays, and non-donor-specific assays, such as spontaneous blastogenesis and autologous mixed lymphocyte reactivity. The phenotypic analysis of peripheral blood lymphocytes, by flow cytometry, and biochemical indices of mononuclear cell metabolism, such as neopterin, procoagulant activity, interleukin 2 receptors and renal tubular antigens, will all be discussed.

While, at a basic science level, these studies have increased our understanding of the mechanisms underlying allograft rejection, it must be stated from the outset that no test yet devised will predict allograft rejection with a sufficient degree of sensitivity and specificity to allow its routine use as a sole clinical test. Nevertheless, the need for such a test remains and continued efforts in this field are required.

IMMUNOLOGICAL MONITORING PRETRANSPLANT
Histocompatibility
HLA

While some controversy remains, more and more studies now show that good HLA matching significantly improves the chances for a successful renal transplant[3–7]. In a small trial in a single centre, Sengar and colleagues showed that matching at HLA-DRW 52/53 and HLA-DQ is an important predictor of allograft survival[5]. The implication of this study was that our priority should be to avoid mismatching at these broad reacting specificities and then to minimize incompatibility at HLA-DR and HLA-B.

In a recent study, Opelz reported that well-matched exchanged kidneys survived better than poorly matched locally transplanted kidneys[6]. Furthermore, Takiff and colleagues have shown that histocompatibility between donor and recipient had by far the greatest influence on the long-term success of renal allografts[7]. Thus, the importance of HLA matching is becoming clear.

Vascular endothelial cells (VEC)

The recognition that rejection may occur even in HLA-identical sibling transplants has led to a search for other antigen systems. One of these (VEC) was noted by Cerilli and colleagues. They found that vascular endothelial cells and monocytes share an antigen system which is highly immunogenic[8]. The major histocompatibility complex is linked with the VEC system. An analysis of crossmatches suggests that a majority of living related allografts may be lost due to pre-sensitization to VEC antigens.

Red blood cell antigens

(1) ABO antigen system
  Compatibility with the ABO blood group system has been considered necessary for a successful renal transplant. This is because AB blood group antigens are present in vascular endothelium.

97

Thus, the crossing of this barrier was thought to lead to hyperacute rejection. However, isolated cases have appeared describing successful transplantation across the ABO barrier[9]. While ABO-mismatched transplants ought to be avoided, one series of patients with liver allografts has been successfully performed across ABO[9]. Rejection was more severe in these cases and occurred earlier, but the results were satisfactory. Recently, Alexandre and Squifflet have reviewed their experience with 23 ABO-mismatched living related kidney transplantations[9]. Eighteen of these allografts were functioning up to five years post-transplant using a very potent immunosuppressive regimen consisting of antilymphocyte globulin, cyclosporin, azathioprine, steroids, piracetam (an anti-platelet agent), plasmapheresis, synthetic substance A or B or both (depending on the incompatibility) and splenectomy.

Another interesting report by Nelson and colleagues[10] describes the successful transplantation of blood group A_2 living related and cadaveric kidneys into blood group O and B patients. Recipients were not pretreated with splenectomy or plasmapheresis. Antirejection prophylaxis consisted of azathioprine, cyclosporin and prednisone and two patients received prophylactic OKT3. Fourteen patients were transplanted: one living related and 13 cadaveric. There was one hyperacute rejection and five episodes of acute cellular rejection of which three were reversed. 10/14 patients have functioning grafts up to 14 months later. Of particular interest was the observation that acute cellular rejection was accompanied by a rise in anti-A_1 antibody of the IgG class. The reasons why grafts from A_2 donors are accepted are not clear but may be a result of low expression of the A antigen on erythrocytes and vascular endothelium.

(2) Cold agglutinins

Renal transplant recipients may have anti-red blood cell autoantibodies which cause agglutination of RBCs at cold temperatures. This may be a cause of immediate graft failure. These antibodies are not of concern at body temperature but the perfused kidney is cold (4–15°C) and cooling of the recipient's blood as it enters the kidney may agglutinate the RBCs. These clumps may cause intravascular clotting and infarction. Schweizer and colleagues have reported successful renal transplantation in the presence of cold agglutinins using a two-minute flush with a warm saline solution[11]. This brief warming seems to prevent agglutination and did not have an adverse effect on graft function.

Presensitization

Anti-idiotypic antibodies

While the presence of preformed antibodies to donor HLA is a contraindication to renal transplantation, historic positive and current serum negative transplants may be successfully performed[12]. In a recent study, Reed and colleagues demonstrated that successful transplantation in patients with preformed antibodies may depend on the presence of anti-anti-HLA antibodies: blocking anti-idiotypic antibodies[13]. Furthermore, certain patients may develop anti-anti-anti-HLA antibodies, which, by their nature, may potentiate the effects of anti-HLA antibodies. In Reed's study, 9/10 patients who tolerated their grafts had anti-idiotypic antibodies at the time of transplantation. Nine of ten patients who rejected their graft had antibodies that potentiated the cytotoxic activity of anti-donor HLA antibodies.

Immunoglobulin class of anti-T cell antibodies

Chapman and colleagues have shown that the class of the antibody producing the positive anti-T cell crossmatch determines the chances for a successful engraftment[14]. Antibodies which undergo reduction with dithiothreitol are of the IgM class and their presence indicates better chances for success since 7/7 grafts performed against an IgG antibody failed.

Methods for the detection of presensitization

A variety of tests have been devised to evaluate the recipient for donor-specific anti-T cell antibodies. The standard NIH test is now well accepted and will predict hyperacute renal transplant failure so that

99

less than 0.5% of renal allografts are lost to this complication[15]. A new method for crossmatching has recently been reported using the flow cytometer and seems to demonstrate an entirely new level of sensitivity and specificity. Garovoy and colleagues showed that there was a much higher incidence of primary non-function in patients with a positive flow cytometry crossmatch than those in whom the test is negative[16]. The cause of graft failure is not classical hyperacute rejection but, nevertheless, a low level of sensitization is detected which leads to non-functional grafts. Terasaki and Cicciarelli have shown that approximately 50 of 200 patients had a positive flow cytometry crossmatch[15]. The non-function rate at one month was 36% in the positive group and 9% in the negative group. Furthermore, in those patients with greater than 10% panel reactivity, 45% had non-function at one month with a positive flow cytometry crossmatch compared with 15% whose test was negative. In addition, in those patients who were retransplanted, 64% had non-function at one month with a positive flow cytometry crossmatch compared with 25% with a negative test. Thus, flow-cytometry crossmatching may help to reduce the incidence of primary non-functioning grafts.

Non-specific lymphocyte reactivity

In a study performed by Langhoff and colleagues[17], recipients of HLA-DR incompatible cadaver kidneys were evaluated for T cell proliferative responses in the presence of phytohaemagglutinin and methylprednisolone. The dose of methylprednisolone required to inhibit proliferation was evaluated pretransplant. They found that patients who required high doses of methylprednisolone had significantly worse one-year graft survival (29%) than those who required low doses (86%) if the patients were treated with azathioprine and steroids. A similar, although not statistically significant, relationship was seen in the cyclosporin group (76% vs. 57%). These data imply that one may predict which patients may receive HLA-DR-incompatible grafts.

IMMUNOLOGIC MONITORING POST-TRANSPLANT

Core biopsies and fine-needle aspiration cytology

One of the most useful and time-proven methods for the diagnosis of rejection has been the standard core biopsy with tissue sections stained with haematoxylin and eosin. The description of this technique is beyond the scope of this manuscript and the reader is referred to two excellent reviews for further information[18,19]. Suffice it to say that core biopsies, while continuing to be the mainstay for diagnosis, do not always correlate with the clinical picture, and each biopsy, even in the most skilled and experienced hands, carries with it a significant, albeit small, risk of morbidity and possibly even graft loss. Thus, there remains a pressing need for the further refinement of diagnostic measures.

One approach has been to evaluate the structure and function of inflammatory cells. In some cases, these studies have taken advantage of recent advances in monoclonal antibody technology, fluorescence activated cell sorter analysis, and techniques of long-term T cell culture. Our laboratory has been evaluating the T cells which infiltrate the rejecting renal allograft by producing long-term T cell lines from minute fragments of tissue[20,21]. We have discovered that T cells obtained in this way are highly specific cytotoxic T cells directed against the alloantigens of the donor of the allograft[20]. Furthermore, we have identified an unusual lymphocyte in the cultures which displays CD4 and CD8 simultaneously[21].

We and others have been looking at the phenotype of the cells which infiltrate the rejecting allograft. These studies reveal that T cells are a major proportion of the graft-infiltrating cells. CD8 + lymphocytes are among the most numerous and macrophages are also well represented[22,23]. The location of the CD8 + cells may also be important as a diffuse cortical distribution may carry a particularly poor prognosis[24]. Another bad prognostic indicator appears to be the presence of a large number of eosinophils in the rejecting allograft[25].

Fine-needle aspiration cytology, as described by Hayry and von Willebrand, has proved to be a significant advance in this field[26]. These biopsies are relatively atraumatic and therefore may be performed daily. Evaluation of the parenchymal component allows for the diagnosis of acute tubular necrosis and cyclosporin nephrotoxicity. Assess-

101

ment of the inflammatory component allows the observation of different patterns of rejection, including the proportions of macrophages, T cells, plasma cells and large granular lymphocytes. Furthermore, expression of HLA class II on renal vascular endothelium may be a good indicator of a rejecting allograft.

Antidonor immune responses

In early studies, we evaluated a variety of immune responses sequentially post-transplant[27] and found that cell-mediated lymphocytotoxicity preceded and accompanied 41/45 rejection episodes. This assay was performed using PHA-activated splenic lymphocytes as the target in standard ^{51}Cr release assays, with ficoll separated mononuclear cells of the recipient as effectors. Complement-dependent antibody also significantly correlated with rejection. This assay was performed using the patient's serum as the source of antibody which fixed rabbit complement and the same splenic lymphocytes were used as targets. Furthermore, a persistently elevated cell-mediated lymphocytotoxicity assay after therapy for rejection predicted re-rejection.

Non-donor-specific lymphocyte reactivity

T Rosette formation and spontaneous blastogenesis

Kerman and colleagues evaluated the presence of active T rosette forming cells and spontaneous blastogenesis in the peripheral blood of renal transplant recipients[28]. They found that a decrease in the rosette forming cells and an increase in spontaneous blastogenesis correlated with rejection, while an increase in rosette forming cells and a decrease in spontaneous blastogenesis correlated with clinical quiescence.

Autologous mixed lymphocyte reaction

The autologous mixed lymphocyte reaction was described by Opelz and colleagues who noted proliferation of T cells in response to large numbers of autologous non-T cells[29]. T cells which proliferate in this reaction demonstrate memory and specificity, and generate cytokines with interleukin 3-like properties[30]. The autologous mixed lymphocyte reaction is, therefore, a good model for the interaction between cells involved in the immune response. The role of the reaction *in vivo* is not clear; however, its absence is associated with profound levels of immunosuppression in renal transplant recipients[31,32].

Antibody-dependent cellular cytotoxicity

Dumble and colleagues evaluated renal transplant recipients for their ability to lyse an antibody-coated cell line (ADCC)[33]. They found that 31/33 rejection episodes were preceded by the presence of ADCC activity 3–5 days prior to clinical diagnosis. In contrast, 6 recipients who did not experience rejection showed no evidence of ADCC activity.

Phenotypic analysis of peripheral blood lymphocytes

Analysis of subset and activation markers

Initial studies by Colvin and colleagues[34,35] suggested that the peripheral blood lymphocyte CD4/CD8 ratio might be of considerable value in HLA non-identical kidney recipients treated with azathioprine and prednisone. Those patients with a ratio > 1 were far more likely to have a rejection episode in the first three months than those who had a ratio < 1. However, those patients who did reject with a low ratio (< 1) had a very poor prognosis regarding rejection reversal. Most patients who had renal allograft dysfunction with a low ratio were found to be infected with a herpes group virus and many had a characteristic form of glomerulopathy[36].

Workers in many centres have analysed the CD4/CD8 ratio, and, to date, over 1000 patients have been reported. Immunosuppressive treatment has varied, and has included either azathioprine and prednisone, with or without antilymphocyte globulin or OKT3, or cyclosporin has been used. Monitoring has been performed with various kinds of flow cytometers. Some of these machines could analyse the buffy coat while others required ficoll-hypaque separation of mononuclear cells. Other groups monitored with simple fluorescence microscopy. A certain degree of agreement exists in the following areas: Most centres, but not all, agree that patients receiving azathioprine and prednisone are more likely to reject with a higher CD4/CD8 ratio[35,37–41]. In other words, patients who reject generally have higher ratios than those patients who maintain stable allograft function. Viral infections are associated with low CD4/CD8 ratios[36,40–42], and renal failure that occurs in the presence of a low CD4/CD8 ratio respond poorly to conventional therapy[35,43]

Significant controversy exists regarding whether the CD4/CD8 ratio rises prior to rejection. Stated in another way, is this parameter predictive? The answer would appear to be no. This is clearly one of the greatest limitations of this index. One is not able to make predictions about individual patients. In any case, as stated by Colvin *et al.*[35], it is remarkable that such crude ratios of T cell subsets, irrespective of their immunologic specificity, often correlate with the activity of renal allograft rejection and other diseases with altered immune function, such as the acquired immune deficiency syndrome (AIDS)[44] and multiple sclerosis[45]. Presumably, one is observing the systemic effects of lymphokines and other mediators which influence overall proliferation and migration of the CD4+ and CD8+ subsets of circulating lymphocytes.

Another approach has been to analyse the lymphocyte cell surface for only those markers which appear with T cell activation. When resting T lymphocytes are exposed to alloantigens, soluble antigens or plant lectins, they undergo a series of changes termed activation. A sequence of events takes place which includes changes in morphology, protein synthesis, cellular proliferation and maturation to a new state of activity. These stages may be identified by analysing various antigenic determinants which appear on these lymphocytes early (< 24 h), with peak cellular proliferation or late. The early stage of activation includes expression of the 4F2 antigen which may be important in Na^+/Ca^{2+} exchange in T cells[46]. Early activation also includes[47] expression of the receptor for interleukin 2 as defined by CD25. The increase in the quantitative expression of CD7 is another early event in T cell activation[48].

The CD38 antigen and the transferrin receptor (TR) appear with peak cellular proliferation[49,50]. CD38 is a marker of the majority of cortical thymocytes and is lost upon maturation. When T lymphocytes are activated, they reacquire CD38. The transferrin receptor is involved in T cell proliferation[51] and may be the target for natural killer cells[52]. Antibodies directed against human Ia-like antigens, such as OKIal, recognize structures which appear late in lectin-stimulated cultures, but with peak cellular proliferation in tetanus toxoid and mixed lymphocyte cultures[49,50]. Antibodies of this type inhibit soluble antigen- and alloantigen-induced activation[53]. Act I is a cell surface antigen which appears 1–2 days after peak cellular proliferation. Act I is a 63 000 dalton polypeptide and is hypothesized to be a marker for maturation and functional activity[54].

In the light of this information, it seems reasonable that the enumeration of lymphocytes expressing activation antigens might assist in the early diagnosis of transplant rejection. Preliminary work from our laboratory (Figure 4.1) suggests that the percentage of peripheral blood lymphocytes and urinary lymphocytes expressing Act I rises in association with rejection (Lazarovits, unpublished). Mohanakumar and colleagues have shown that transferrin receptors behave in the same manner[55]. On the other hand, infection also seems to cause an increase in cell activation antigen expression. Thus, specificity remains a problem. Perhaps elevated transferrin receptors associated with a low CD4/CD8 ratio might indicate activation from infection rather than rejection.

The effects of immunotherapy on the phenotypic analysis of peripheral blood lymphocytes

Using monoclonal antibodies and flow cytometry, one may monitor the effects of various treatment regimens on peripheral blood lymphocytes. Corticosteroids have been shown to reduce transiently the number of CD4+ lymphocytes[56]. Cyclosporin has little acute effect on the number of circulating T cells, but after about two months, the

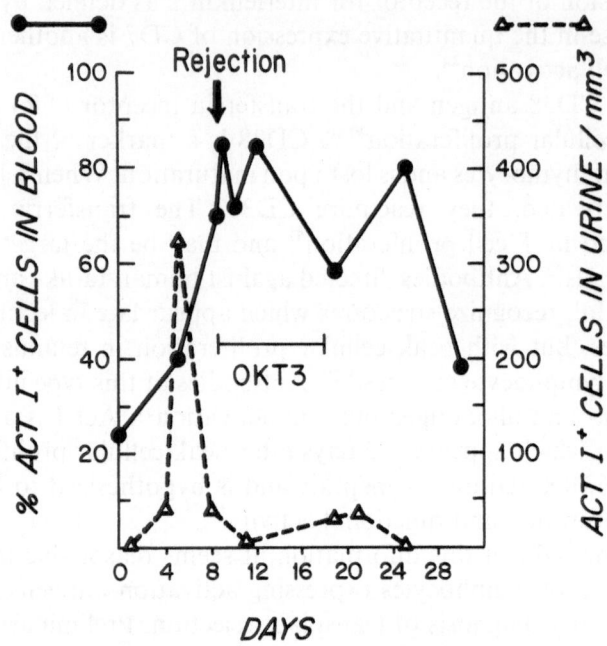

FIGURE 4.1 Sequential enumeration of peripheral blood lymphocytes and urinary lymphocytes using anti-Act I monoclonal antibody[54,65]. OKT3 was started on day 9. The number of Act I+ cells rose in both the peripheral blood and urine in the days preceding the diagnosis

number of circulating CD8+ cells is often increased[57]. Low doses of cyclophosphamide tend to decrease the number of CD4+ cells[56]. Thoracic duct drainage[58], total lymphoid irradiation[59] and anti-lymphocyte globulin[34] therapy all produce a prolonged depression of CD4+ cells, while the CD8+ cells regenerate more quickly.

Recently, rejection therapy has been specifically targeted towards the T cell using the murine monoclonal antibody OKT3[34,60]. This antibody clusters with CD3 which consists of five chains 20–26 kilodaltons of relative molecular mass in association with two variable immunoglobulin-like glycoproteins which form the T lymphocyte antigen receptor (CD3-Ti)[61]. OKT3 has profound effects on T cell function *in vitro*. First of all it removes CD3-Ti from the lymphocyte cell surface: a phenomenon termed modulation[34]. This prevents allo-specific cytotoxicity[62] as well as induction of proliferation *in vitro*[63]. The exact mechanism by which OKT3 reverses rejection is not clear; however, much information is expected from a recently published animal model[64]. What is clear is that OKT3 eliminates peripheral blood T cells from the circulation within minutes of injection. As shown in Figure 4.2, over the days following OKT3 therapy, the peripheral blood T cells return to the circulation but they lack CD3-Ti. Other surface markers, such as CD7, are present. As long as CD3-Ti remains absent, rejection is unlikely to recur, although two cases have documented the recurrence of rejection in the absence of CD3 + lymphocytes[65]. This is certainly a rare occurrence. On the other hand, antimurine antibodies develop frequently in patients receiving OKT3[66]. If the antibody response is against the idiotype, the OKT3 is eliminated from the blood. Should this occur, as in Figure 4.2, then the surface of the cell re-expresses CD3-Ti as measured by the flow cytometer. Rejection may recur if the re-expression goes unrecognized. Monitoring of surface expression of CD3-Ti will become even more important as patients receive a subsequent course in OKT3 where the danger of an anti-idiotypic response is even greater.

Long-term renal allograft recipients are at increased risk of developing cancers and chronic infections compared with normal individuals. One possible explanation for this phenomenon has been proposed by Legendre and colleagues[67]. They have found an expanded large granular lymphocyte subset which lacks natural killer activity in these patients. The presence of a large percentage of these CD3 +, Leu7 +, CD16 − cells may be a marker for the chronically immuno-depressed state.

Analysis of mononuclear cell metabolism

Neopterin

This substance is derived from guanosine triphosphate. Its excretion in the urine and concentration in the serum is elevated in rare cases of phenylketonuria and in conditions characterized by hyperactivity of the cellular immune system[68,69]. The pathway for neopterin release by macrophages requires T cell activation and the production of γ-

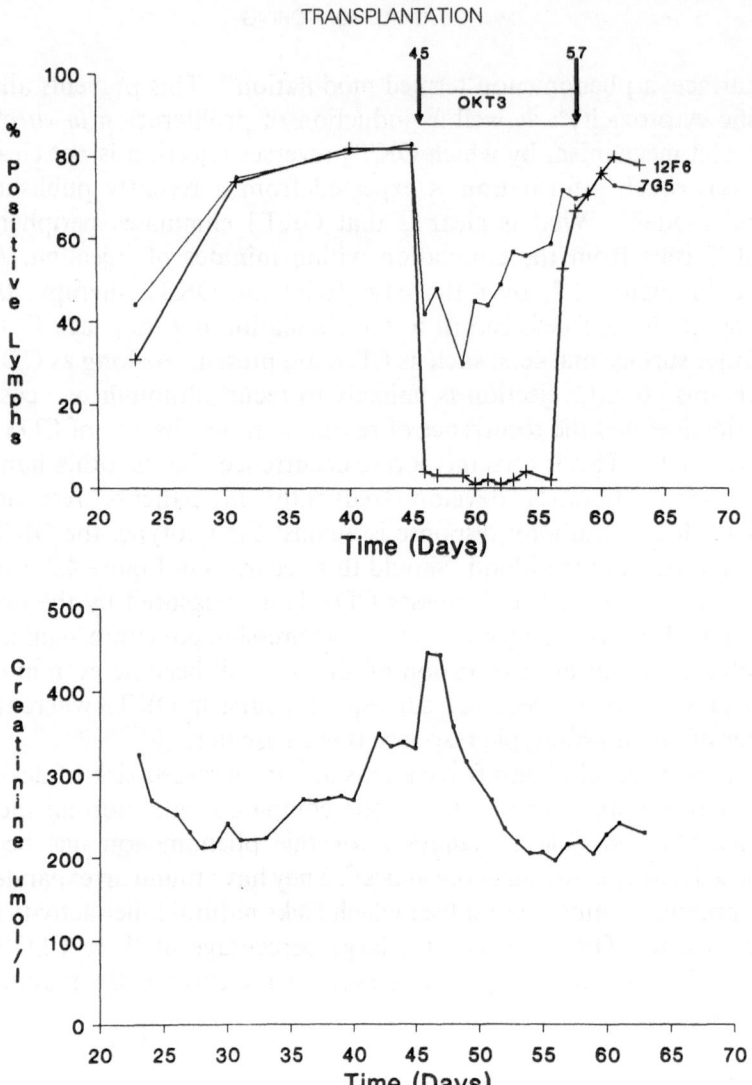

FIGURE 4.2   Sequential enumeration of peripheral blood lymphocytes using 12F6 (CD3) and 7G5 (CD7) monoclonal antibodies[65]. OKT3 was started on day 45, with resolution of symptoms by day 49. Concomitant medication consisted of prednisone and azathioprine. Anti-OKT3 antibodies developed by day 57, and were manifested by a return of 12F6 (CD3) expression on the peripheral blood lymphocytes. Cyclosporin was therefore recommenced, the OKT3 was discontinued, and the patient has remained free of rejection

interferon. Margreiter and colleagues evaluated urinary neopterin excretion in renal transplant recipients. They found that major immunological complications, such as rejection and viral infections, were frequently preceded by high or rising neopterin levels[68]. Similarly, plasma neopterin levels rose in a study by Schafer and colleagues[69].

Procoagulant activity

Monocytes are involved in allograft rejection through a variety of pathways, including delayed type hypersensitivity. Monocytes release an activity termed procoagulant after triggering by T cells through an interaction which is MHC restricted. The presence of the procoagulant activity is of interest because it links cell-mediated immunity and the coagulation system in an antigen-specific way[70,71]. The procoagulant activity was measured in two studies[70,71] which demonstrated a rise prior to the diagnosis of rejection in a significant number of cases. However, procoagulant activity was also high immediately post-transplant, indicating that it is not specific for rejection; in spite of this, it may be a useful adjunct in the clinical management of these patients.

Interleukin 2 receptors

Release of interleukin 2 receptors (IL2R) into the supernatant by activated T cells *in vitro* is among the earliest events during T cell activation. Colvin and colleagues[72] found that elevated levels of IL2R occurred in acute cellular rejection but were not similarly increased in acute renal failure from non-immunologic causes, such as cyclosporin nephrotoxicity, renal artery stenosis and haemolytic–uraemic syndrome. IL2R were also elevated during viral infections and during treatment for rejection with monoclonal and polyclonal anti-lymphocyte antibodies.

Analysis of renal tubular antigens

Shen and colleagues have prepared a murine monoclonal antibody which identifies an epithelial surface antigen in human renal proximal tubules[73]. They evaluated serum levels of this antigen (HRTE) and found a two-fold increase in 56/62 rejection episodes 2–5 days before the clinical diagnosis was made. Furthermore, the HRTE level fell toward normal with successful treatment with steroids but remained elevated in the steroid-resistant rejection episodes. However, cyclosporin nephrotoxicity also produced a similar increase in HRTE levels with a concomitant decrease as the nephrotoxicity resolved with reduced dosage.

Tolkoff-Rubin and colleagues utilized two murine monoclonal antibodies (URO-4 and URO-4a) directed against different epitopes of the adenosine-deaminase-binding protein (ABP) for detection of ABP in the urine[74]. 29/29 acute rejection episodes had elevated ABP levels 1–7 days before the treatment commenced. Those whose level fell to normal during therapy had successful reversal. On the other hand, 10/12 whose ABP level remained elevated had re-rejection within 7 days of completion of therapy. However, cyclosporin nephrotoxicity also produced high ABP levels in the urine.

Prolactin

Prolactin receptors have been identified on human T and B lymphocytes[75]. Furthermore, cyclosporin seems to prevent the binding of prolactin to these receptors[75]. It is, therefore, of interest that Carrier and colleagues demonstrated a rise in serum prolactin 6–8 days prior to every first episode of rejection in their cardiac allograft recipients[76]. There were, however, a number of false positives which affected the value of the test.

CONCLUSIONS

One of the goals of immunological monitoring in clinical medicine is to allow for the optimization of immunotherapy. This involves the selection of donor–recipient pairs which will decrease the risk of rejection and the accurate differentiation between rejection, infection, cyclosporin nephrotoxicity and acute tubular necrosis as the cause of renal allograft dysfunction, which are the major diagnostic dilemmas. Thus, patients who are undergoing rejection will not have the cyclosporin dose decreased, thereby worsening the rejection activity, because of a misdiagnosis. Furthermore, patients with acute tubular necrosis will not receive unnecessary doses of methylprednisolone or monoclonal antibody, when all that was needed was time and patience. Those patients who do undergo rejection will receive an optimum amount of immunotherapy: one hopes for enough to establish immunological quiescence and not so much that infections develop.

If this goal could be met, then transplant patients would have a better chance of keeping their grafts and they would have a decreased incidence of morbidity and mortality. Much work remains since no test yet devised can claim success. Nevertheless, the field of immunological monitoring may one day form an integral and productive component in the clinical management of a transplant patient.

Acknowledgements

This work was supported in part by grants from the Physicians' Services Incorporated Foundation and the Kidney Foundation of Canada.

We thank M. White, C. Henderson and J. Yamada for their excellent technical assistance, and K. McCormick for the typing of the manuscript.

REFERENCES

1. Stiller, C. R., Robinette, M. A. and Dyer, A. (1985). Organ donors in the eighties: The minister's task force on kidney donation. *Transplant. Proc.*, **17**, 5–8

2. Canadian Multicentre Transplant Study Group (1986). A randomized clinical trial of cyclosporine in cadaveric renal transplantation: Analysis at three years. *N. Engl. J. Med.*, **314**, 1219–1225

3. Sanfilippo, F., Vaughn, W. K., Spees, E. K., Light, J. A. and LeFor, W. M. (1984). Benefits of HLA-A and HLA-B matching on graft and patient outcome after cadaveric-donor renal transplantation. *N. Engl. J. Med.*, **311**, 358–364

4. Opelz, G. (1985). Correlation of HLA matching with kidney graft survival in patients with or without cyclosporine treatment. *Transplantation*, **40**, 240–242

5. Sengar, D. P. S., Couture, R. A., Raman, S., Jindal, S. L. and Lazarovits, A. I. (1987). Role of class I and class II HLA antigens in cadaveric renal transplantation. *Transplant. Proc.*, **19**, 3422–3425

6. Opelz, G. (1988). The benefit of exchanging donor kidneys among transplant centers. *N. Engl. J. Med.*, **318**, 1289–1294

7. Takiff, H., Cook, D. J., Himaya, N. S., Mickey, M. R. and Terasaki, P. I. (1988). Dominant effect of histocompatibility on ten-year kidney transplant survival. *Transplantation*, **45**, 410–415

8. Cerilli, J., Brasile, L., Galouzis, T., Lempert, N. and Clarke, J. (1985). The vascular endothelial cell antigen system. *Transplantation*, **39**, 286–289

9. Alexandre, G. P. J. and Squifflet, J. P. (1988). Significance of the ABO antigen system. In Cerilli, G. J. (ed.) *Organ Transplantation and Replacement*, pp. 223–230. (Philadelphia: J. P. Lippincott Company)

10. Nelson, P. W., Helling, T. S., Pierce, G. E., Ross, G., Shield, C. F., Beck, M. L., Blake, B. and Cross, D. E. (1988). Successful transplantation of blood group A_2 kidneys into non-A recipients. *Transplantation*, **45**, 316–319

11. Schweizer, R. T., Bartus, S. A., Perkins, H. A. and Belzer, F. O. (1982). Renal allograft failure and cold red blood cell autoagglutinins. *Transplantation*, **33**, 77–79

12. Cardella, C. J., Falk, J. A., Nicholson, M. J., Harding, M. and Cook, G. T. (1982). Successful renal transplantation in patients with T-cell reactivity to donor. *Lancet*, **2**, 1240–1243

13. Reed, E., Hardy, M., Benvenisty, A., Lattes, C., Brensilver, J., McCabe, R., Reemstma, K., King, D. W. and Suciu-Foca, N. (1987). Effect of antiidiotypic antibodies to HLA on graft survival in renal-allograft recipients. *N. Engl. J. Med.*, **316**, 1450–1455

14. Chapman, J. R., Taylor, C. J., Ting, A. and Morris, P. J. (1986). Immunoglobulin class and specificity of antibodies causing positive T cell crossmatches: Relationship to renal transplant outcome. *Transplantation*, **42**, 608–613

15. Terasaki, P. I. and Cicciarelli, J. (1988). Sensitization and its role in transplantation. In Cerilli, G. J. (ed.) *Organ Transplantation and Replacement*, pp. 196–207. (Philadelphia: J. B. Lippincott Company)

16. Garovoy, M. R., Colombe, B. W., Melzer, J., Feduska, N., Shields, C., Cross, D., Amend, W., Vincenti, F., Hopper, S., Duca, R. and Salvatierra, O. (1985). Flow cytometry crossmatching for donor-specific transfusion recipients and cadaveric transplantation. *Transplant. Proc.*, **17**, 693–695

17. Langhoff, E., Ladefoged, J., Jakobsen, B. K., Platz, P., Ryder, L. P., Svejgaard, A. and Thaysen, J. H. (1986). Recipient lymphocyte sensitivity to methylprednisolone affects cadaver kidney graft survival. *Lancet*, **2**, 1296–1297

18. Porter, K. A. (1983). Renal transplantation. In Heptinstall, R. H. (ed.) *Pathology of the Kidney*, pp. 1455–1547 (Boston: Little, Brown and Company)

19. Olsen, T. S. (1986). Pathology of allograft rejection. In Williams, G. M., Burdick, J. F. and Solez, K. (eds.) *Kidney Transplant Rejection*, pp. 173–197. (New York: Marcel Dekker, Inc.)

20. Mayer, T. G., Fuller, A. A., Fuller, T. C., Lazarovits, A. I., Boyle, L. A. and Kurnick, J. T. (1985). Characterization of *in vivo* activated allospecific T lymphocytes propagated from human renal allograft biopsies undergoing rejection. *J. Immunol.*, **134**, 258–264

21. Preffer, F. I., Colvin, R. B., Leary, C. P., Boyle, L. A., Tuazon, T. V., Lazarovits, A. I., Cosimi, A. B. and Kurnick, J. T. (1986). Two colour flow cytometry and functional analysis of lymphocytes cultured from human renal allografts: identification of a Leu 2 + 3 + subpopulation. *J. Immunol.*, **137**, 2823–2830

22. Platt, J. L., LeBien, T. W. and Michael, A. F. (1982). Interstitial mononuclear cell populations in renal graft rejection: Identification by monoclonal antibodies in tissue sections. *J. Exp. Med.*, **155**, 17–30

23. Hancock, W. W., Thomson, N. M. and Atkins, R. C. (1983). Composition of interstitial cellular infiltrate identified by monoclonal antibodies in renal biopsies of rejecting human renal allografts. *Transplantation*, **35**, 458–463

24. Sanfilippo, F., Kolbeck, P. C., Vaughn, W. K. and Bollinger, R. R. (1985). Renal allograft cell infiltrates associated with irreversible rejection. *Transplantation*, **40**, 679–684

25. Weir, M. R., Hall-Craggs, M., Shen, S. Y., Posner, J. N., Alongi, S. V., Dagher, F. J. and Sadler, J. H. (1986). The prognostic value of the eosinophil in acute renal allograft rejection. *Transplantation*, **41**, 709–712

26. Hayry, P. J. and von Willebrand, E. (1986). Aspiration cytology in monitoring human allografts. In Williams, G. M., Burdick, J. F. and Solez, K. (eds.) *Kidney Transplant Rejection*, pp. 247–262. (New York: Marcel Dekker, Inc.)

27. Stiller, C. R., Sinclair, N. R., Abrahams, S., McGirr, D., Singh, H., Howson, W. T. and Ulan, R. A. (1976). Anti-donor immune responses in prediction of transplant rejection. *N. Engl. J. Med.*, **294**, 978–982

28. Kerman, R. H., Floyd, M., Van Buren, C., McConnell, B. J., McConnell, R. and Kahan, B. D. (1981). Correlation of nonspecific immune monitoring with rejection or impaired function of renal allografts. *Transplantation*, **32**, 16–23

29. Opelz, G., Kiuchi, M., Takasugi, M. and Terasaki, P. I. (1975). Autologous stimulation of human lymphocyte subpopulations. *J. Exp. Med.*, **142**, 1327–1332

30. Suzuki, R., Suzuki, S., Takahashi, T. and Kumagai, K. (1986). Production of a cytokine with interleukin 3 like properties and cytokine-dependent proliferation in human autologous mixed lymphocyte reaction. *J. Exp. Med.*, **164**, 1682–1699

31. Fuller, L., Flaa, C., Jaffe, D., Strauss, J., Kyriakides, G. K. and Miller, J. (1983). Factors affecting the autologous mixed lymphocyte reaction in kidney transplantation. *J. Clin. Invest.*, **71**, 1322–1330

32. Fuller, L., Esquenazi, V., Roth, D., Milgrom, M., Haynes, M. and Miller, J. (1987). The clinical significance of the autologous mixed lymphocyte reaction in transplantation. *Transplant. Proc.*, **19**, 1562–1563

33. Dumble, L. J., Macdonald, I. M. and Kincaid-Smith, P. (1980). Human renal allograft rejection is predicted by serial determinations of antibody-dependent cellular cytotoxicity. *Transplantation*, **29**, 30–34

34. Cosimi, A. B., Colvin, R. B., Burton, R. C., Rubin, R. H., Goldstein, G., Kung, P. C., Hansen, W. P., Delmonico, F. L. and Russell, P. S. (1981). Use of monoclonal antibodies to T-cell subsets for immunologic monitoring and treatment in

recipients of renal allografts. *N. Engl. J. Med.*, **305**, 308–314
35. Colvin, R. B., Cosimi, A. B., Burton, R. C., Delmonico, F. L., Jaffers, G., Rubin, R. H., Tolkoff-Rubin, N. E., Giorgi, J. V., McCluskey, R. T. and Russell, P. S. (1983). Circulating T-cell subsets in 72 human renal allograft recipients: The OKT4⁺/OKT8⁺ cell ratio correlates with reversibility of graft injury and glomerulopathy. *Transplant. Proc.*, **15**, 1166–1169
36. Schooley, R. T., Hirsch, M. S., Colvin, R. B., Cosimi, A. B., Tolkoff-Rubin, N. E., McCluskey, R. T., Burton, R. C., Russell, P. S., Herrin, J. T., Delmonico, F. L., Giorgi, J. V., Henle, W. and Rubin, R. H. (1983). Association of herpes virus infections with T-lymphocyte-subset alterations, glomerulopathy, and opportunistic infections afer renal transplantation. *N. Engl. J. Med.*, **308**, 307–313
37. Smith, W. J., Burdick, J. F. and Williams, G. M. (1983). Immunologic monitoring of renal transplant recipients. *Transplant. Proc*, **15**, 1182–1183
38. Binkley, W. F., Valenzuela, R., Braun, W. E., Deodhar, S. D., Novick, A. C. and Steinmuller, D. R. (1983). Flow cytometry quantitation of peripheral blood (PB) T-cell subsets in human renal allograft recipients. *Transplant. Proc.*, **15**, 1163–1165
39. Carter, N. P., Cullen, P. R., Thompson, J. F., Bewick, A. L. T., Wood, R. F. M. and Morris, P. J. (1983). Monitoring lymphocyte subpopulations in renal allograft recipients., *Transplant. Proc.*, **15**, 1157–1159
40. Chatenoud, L., Chkoff, N., Kreis, H. and Bach, J. F. (1983). Correlation between immunoregulatory T-cell imbalances and renal allograft outcome. *Transplant Proc.*, **15**, 1184–1185
41. Guttmann, R. D. and Poulsen, R. S. (1983). Fluorescence activated cell sorter analysis of lymphocyte subsets after renal transplantation. *Transplant. Proc.*, **15**, 1160–1162
42. Shen, S. Y., Weir, M. R., Kosenko, A., Revie, D. R., Ordonez, J. V., Dagher, F. J., Chretien, P. and Sadler, J. H. (1985). Reevaluation of T cell subset monitoring in cyclosporine-treated renal allograft recipients. *Transplantation*, **40**, 620–622
43. Van Es, A., Tanke, H. J., Baldwin, W. M., Oljans, P. J., Ploem, J. S. and Van Es, L. A. (1983). Ratios of T lymphocyte subpopulations predict survival of cadaveric renal allografts in adult patients on low dose corticosteroid therapy. *Clin. Exp. Immunol.*, **52**, 13–20
44. Fahey, J. L., Prince, H., Weaver, M., Groopman, J., Visscher, B., Schwartz, K. and Detels, R. (1984). Quantitative changes in T helper or T suppressor/cytotoxic lymphocyte subsets that distinguish acquired immune deficiency syndrome from other immune subset disorders. *Am. J. Med.*, **76**, 95–100
45. Reinherz, E. L., Weiner, H. L., Hauser, S. L., Cohen, J. A., Distaso, J. A. and Schlossman, S. F. (1980). Loss of suppressor T cells in active multiple sclerosis. *N. Engl. J. Med.*, **303**, 125–129
46. Bron, C., Rousseaux, M., Spiazzi, A. and MacDonald, H. R. (1986). Structural homology between the human 4F2 antigen and a murine cell surface glycoprotein associated with lymphocyte activation. *J. Immunol.*, **137**, 397–399
47. Uchiyama, T., Broder, S. and Waldmann, T. A. (1981). A monoclonal antibody (anti-Tac) reactive with activated and functionally mature human T cells. *J. Immunol.*, **126**, 1393–1397
48. Lazarovits, A. I., Colvin, R. B., Camerini, D., Karsh, J. and Kurnick, J. T. (1987). Modulation of CD7 is associated with T lymphocyte function. In McMichael, A. (ed.) *Leucocyte Typing III*, pp. 219–223. (Oxford: Oxford University Press)

49. Cotner, T., Williams, J. M., Christenson, L., Shapiro, H. M., Strom, T. B. and Strominger, J. (1983). Simultaneous flow cytometric analysis of human T cell activation antigen expression and DNA content. *J. Exp. Med.*, **157**, 461–472

50. Hercend, T., Ritz, J., Schlossman, S. F. and Reinherz, E. L. (1981). Comparative expression of T9, T10, and Ia antigens on activated human T cell subsets. *Hum. Immunol.*, **3**, 247–259

51. Mendelsohn, J., Trowbridge, I. and Castagnola, J. (1983). Inhibition of human lymphocyte proliferation by monoclonal antibody to transferrin receptor. *Blood*, **62**, 821–826

52. Vodinelich, L., Sutherland, R., Schneider, C., Newman, R. and Greaves, M. (1983). Receptor for transferrin may be a 'target' structure for natural killer cells. *Proc. Natl. Acad. Sci. USA*, **80**, 835–839

53. Koide, Y., Awashima, F., Yoshida, T. O., Takenouchi, T., Wakisaka, A., Moriuchi, J. and Aizawa, M. (1982). The role of three distinct Ia-like antigen molecules in human T cell proliferative responses: Effect of monoclonal anti-Ia-like antibodies. *J. Immunol.*, **129**, 1061–1069

54. Lazarovits, A. I., Moscicki, R. A., Kurnick, J. T., Camerini, D., Bhan, A. K., Baird, L. G., Erikson, M. and Colvin, R. B. (1984). Lymphocyte activation antigens. I. A monoclonal antibody, anti-Act I, defines a new late lymphocyte activation antigen. *J. Immunol.*, **133**, 1857–1862

55. Mohanakumar, T., Hoshinaga, K., Wood, N. L., Szentpetery, S. and Lower, R. R. (1986). Enumeration of transferrin-receptor-expressing lymphocytes as a potential marker for rejection in human cardiac transplant recipients. *Transplantation*, **42**, 691–694

56. Bast, R. C., Reinherz, E. L., Maver, C., Lavin, P. and Schlossman, S. F. (1983). Contrasting effects of cyclophosphamide and prednisolone on the phenotype of human peripheral blood leukocytes. *Clin. Immunol. Immunopathol.*, **28**, 101–114

57. Sweny, P. and Tidman, N. (1982). The effect of cyclosporin A on peripheral blood T cell subpopulations in renal allografts. *Clin. Exp. Immunol.*, **47**, 445–448

58. Laville, M., Cordier, G., Brochier, J., Lefebvre, R., Revillard, J. P. and Traeger, J. (1982). Improvement of cadaveric renal allograft survival by thoracic duct drainage: Relation with T-lymphocyte subset modifications assessed by flow-cytometry. *Proc. Eur. Dial. Transplant. Assoc.*, **19**, 488–494

59. Kotzin, B. L., Kansas, G. S. Engleman, E. G., Hoppe, R. T., Kaplan, H. S. and Strober, S. (1983). Changes in T-cell subsets in patients with rheumatoid arthritis treated with total lymphoid irradiation. *Clin. Immunol. Immunopathol.*, **27**, 250–260

60. Ortho Multicenter Transplant Study Group (1985). A randomized clinical trial of OKT3 monoclonal antibody for acute rejection of cadaveric renal transplants. *N. Engl. J. Med.*, **313**, 337–342

61. Weissman, A. M., Samelson, L. E. and Klausner, R. D. (1986). A new subunit of the human T-cell antigen receptor complex. *Nature (London)*, **324**, 480–482

62. Meuer, S. C., Fitzgerald, K. A., Hussey, R. E., Hodgdon, J. C., Schlossman, S. F. and Reinherz, E. L. (1983). Clonotypic structures involved in antigen-specific human T cell function: Relationship to the T3 molecular complex. *J. Exp. Med.*, **157**, 705–719

63. Tax, W. J. M., Willems, H. W., Reekers, P. P. M., Capel, P. J. A. and Koene, R. A. P. (1983). Polymorphism in mitogenic effect of IgG1 monoclonal antibodies against T3 antigen on human T cells. *Nature (London)*, **304**, 445–447

64. Hirsch, R., Eckhaus, M., Auchincloss, H., Sachs, D. H. and Bluestone, J. A. (1988). Effects of in vivo administration of anti-T3 monoclonal antibody on T cell function in mice: I. Immunosuppression of transplantation responses. *J. Immunol.*, **140**, 3766–3772

65. Lazarovits, A. I. and Shield, C. (1988). Recurrence of acute rejection in the absence of CD3 positive lymphocytes. *Clin. Immunol. Immunopathol.* (In press)

66. Jaffers, G. J., Fuller, T. C., Cosimi, A. B., Russell, P. S., Winn, H. J. and Colvin, R. B. (1986). Monoclonal antibody therapy: Anti-idiotypic and non-anti-idiotypic antibodies to OKT3 arising despite intense immunosuppression. *Transplantation*, **41**, 572–578

67. Legendre, C. M., Yip, G. H., Rodrigues, G. A., Forbes, C. and Guttmann, R. D. (1987). Characterization of an expanded large granular lymphocyte subset lacking natural killer activity present in renal allograft recipients. *Transplantation*, **43**, 229–234

68. Margreiter, R., Fuchs, D., Hausen, A., Huber, C., Reibnegger, G., Spielberger, M. and Wachter, H. (1983). Neopterin as a new biochemical marker for diagnosis of allograft rejection: Experience based upon evaluation of 100 consecutive cases. *Transplantation*, **36**, 650–653

69. Schafer, A. J., Daniel, V., Dreikorn, K. and Opelz, G. (1986). Assessment of plasma neopterin in clinical kidney transplantation. *Transplantation*, **41**, 454–459

70. Halloran, P. F., Aprile, M. A., Haddad, G. J. and Robinette, M. A. (1985). Procoagulant activity in renal transplant recipients. *Transplantation*, **39**, 374–377

71. Cole, E. H., Cardella, C. J., Schulman, J. and Levy, G. A. (1985). Monocyte procoagulant activity and plasminogen activator: Role in human renal allograft rejection. *Transplantation*, **40**, 363–371

72. Colvin, R. B., Fuller, T. C., MacKeen, L., Kung, P. C., Ip, S. H. and Cosimi, A. B. (1987). Plasma interleukin 2 receptor levels in renal allograft recipients. *Clin. Immunol. Immunopathol.*, **43**, 273–276

73. Shen, S. Y., Weir, M. R., Litkowski, L., Anthony, R., Welik, R., Kosenko, A., Light, P. D., Dagher, F. J. and Sadler, J. H. (1985). Enzyme-linked immunosorbent assay for serum renal tubular antigen in kidney transplant patients. *Transplantation*, **40**, 642–647

74. Tolkoff-Rubin, N. E., Cosimi, A. B., Delmonico, F. L., Russell, P. S., Thompson, R. E., Piper, D. J., Hansen, W. P., Bander, N. H., Finstad, C. L., Cordon-Cardo, C., Klotz, L. H., Old, L. J. and Rubin, R. H. (1986). Diagnosis of tubular injury in renal transplant patients by a urinary assay for a proximal tubular antigen, the adenosine-deaminase-binding protein. *Transplantation*, **41**, 593–596

75. Russell, D. H., Kibler, R., Matrisian, L., Larson, D. F., Poulos, B. and Magun, B. E. (1985). Prolactin receptors on human T and B lymphocytes: Antagonism of prolactin binding by cyclosporine. *J. Immunol.*, **134**, 3027–3031

76. Carrier, M., Emery, R. W., Wild-Mobley, J., Perrotta, N. J., Russell, D. H. and Copeland, J. G. (1987). Prolactin as a marker of rejection in human heart transplantation. *Transplant. Proc.*, **19**, 3442–3443

5
IMMUNOSUPPRESSION

D. J. G. WHITE, P. FRIEND and R. Y. CALNE

THE IMMUNOLOGY OF GRAFT REJECTION

The rejection of organs transplanted between mismatched individuals of the same species (termed an allograft) represents a unique position in the repertoire of immune responses and is unlike the immune response to any other foreign antigen. The immune activity induced by an allograft represents a specific commitment of the immune system estimated at between 2–10% of the total T cell pool[1]. This probably occurs because the immune system is committed to the recognition of self-histocompatibility antigens (MHC) and responding to these products when they become 'altered' by the presence of a foreign antigen (termed MHC restriction)[2]. The presence as a result of a transplant of foreign MHC antigens causes confusion within the immune system, resulting in an overwhelming response. The exact nature of this immune confusion is currently the subject of much immunological research[3].

In addition to the privileged status of the 'transplantation antigens' in immunology, the exact mechanism by which graft rejection can occur is not fully resolved. It is known that graft rejection is dependent upon thymus-derived cells since T cell-deprived animals (which can, nevertheless, still produce antibody) fail to reject transplants. The recent experiments of Dallman and Mason[4] have shown the overwhelming importance of T helper cells in mediating graft rejection but failed to confirm the effector cell population as being cytotoxic T cells. It seems probable that graft destruction may result from a combined assault by cytotoxic T cells, natural killer cells, lymphokines and other immune activities collectively described as delayed-type hypersensitivity.

Thus, the transplant surgeon is faced with controlling an immune response which is several orders of magnitude greater than that induced by any other primary antigenic stimulus. The process by which this response is induced is unclear and the effector cell mechanism which ultimately destroys the graft is poorly defined. It is perhaps somewhat surprising that any successful cadaveric transplants can be performed. That transplantation is now regarded as a successful therapy for a variety of end-stage organ failures is, in large part, due to the empirical development of the variety of immunosuppressive regimes currently deployed in the clinical practice of organ transplantation.

IRRADIATION AS AN IMMUNOSUPPRESSANT

The first attempts at preventing graft rejection were made by using whole-body irradiation to control the immune system. These attempts[5] demonstrated immediately the fundamental principles involved in immunosuppression. If the potential recipient was given sufficient irradiation to eradicate the immune system, graft rejection was prevented and the recipient invariably died, despite a functioning graft, of overwhelming infection. When the dose of irradiation was reduced to allow a protective remnant of immune function, the graft was then rejected by this remaining immunity. With the advent of pharmacological immunosuppression, irradiation as a means of controlling the immune system fell into disrepute and, for almost two decades, no attempts were made to immunosuppress patients by irradiation.

Recently, however, interest in irradiation as a mechanism for controlling graft rejection has been revived by a series of observations by Slavin et al.[6] Most cells killed by ionizing irradiation die as a result of lesions produced in nucleic acids which cause death during attempted mitotic division. Many of these radiation-induced lesions can be repaired by the action of enzymes in advance of any attempted cell division. It should be stressed that radiation damages all molecules indiscriminately and has no selective effect on DNA. It is the unique role of DNA in cell replication that confers a particular significance to radiation-induced lesions within it. There are, however, in the body, some cells which are highly radiosensitive, including the small resting lymphocyte which dies as a result of radiation damage during interphase. Thus, when radiation doses are fractionated over several days, repair processes can occur in most cells between successive exposures as a result of enzyme activity on the damaged DNA. In the radiosensitive cell population, no such repair occurs and an almost linear dose–response curve can be achieved with this fractionation treatment. It was as a result of this peculiar radiosensitivity of the small lymphocyte that the treatment by fractionation radiation therapy of Hodgkin's disease has proved to be such an effective procedure. It was discovered that, by subjecting involved lymph nodes to a total dose of approximately 4000 rad, given as a fractionated treatment, the disease could be eradicated from those lymph nodes with a recurrence rate of less than 1%. The necessity of treating all involved lymph nodes resulted in the enlargement of the field of exposure by the use of the inverted Y mantle. It was found that most patients could tolerate these very high cumulative doses of such 'total lymphoid irradiation' (TLI) remarkably well.

There has been little clinical evidence that patients treated with TLI for Hodgkin's disease have any impairment of their immune function. There is no long-term evidence of discernible increase in the incidence of infection in this patient population. However, it was demonstrated that these patients had severe and substantial deficiencies in their T cell function. They have a T lymphocytopenia and a B lymphocytosis, depression of responsivenes in mixed lymphocyte cultures and PHA mytogenesis and a loss of delayed-type hypersensitivity responses to rechallenge with skin-sensitivity agents[7]. It was these observations that led Slavin et al.[6] to consider the use of TLI as an immunosuppressive agent in transplantation.

The initial experiments which showed TLI to be immunosuppressive in transplantation were performed using skin grafts between H2-incompatible strains of mice. These studies were then extended to the rat, given either a skin graft or a heart graft. It is perhaps not surprising that a total cumulative dose of more than 3000 rad should prove to be immunosuppressive. However, a remarkable observation was made in further experiments[8] in that it was possible to establish chimeras by

119

the transfer of fully allogeneic bone marrow cells without any indication of the occurrence of subsequent graft versus host disease (GVH). Since GVH is fundamentally a property of the transferred donor cells which, of course, have not been treated in any way, this observation suggests that much of the subsequent clinical condition normally associated with the graft versus host disease must, in practice, rely on a participation of host-controlled factors, Slavin and his colleagues have suggested that the TLI treatment alters the structure of the reticuloendothelial and lymphoid tissues. These changes allow the tolerance of residual host lymphocytes to transplantation antigens from the graft to be established and inhibit the proper maturation of the cells derived from the transplanted bone marrow.

It is clear from these experimental studies that TLI induces some fundamental modification of the immune system and it may well be that the clinical application of this technique could be applied to the induction of chimerism and tolerance for organ grafting of the future. The clinical use of TLI for organ transplantation is, however, currently hampered by several practical considerations. The most pressing of these is the relationship of the timing between the fractionated doses and the availability of an appropriate organ for grafting. This problem is aggravated since the immunosuppressive potency of TLI is currently considered of most value for the treatment of individuals who have previously rejected kidney grafts, thus demonstrating a highly active responder status[9]. Such individuals will often have produced antibodies against a variety of different HLA antigens. The administration of the TLI regime with 200–300 rad fractionated doses takes 2–3 weeks to complete, at which time a search can begin for a crossmatch-negative kidney. Animal studies have shown that there is a critical time period of no more than a few weeks between the last dose of irradiation and the time at which transplantation must take place. Thus, those patients for whom it is difficult to find a suitable crossmatch cytotoxic-negative transplant may require a substantial number of 'topping-up' irradiation treatments. The correct protocols, immunological consequences and side-effects of such topping-up treatments have yet to be fully established. It is clear, however, that such treatments result in potential recipients being given very high cumulative doses of irradiation while waiting for a transplant.

A second consideration for the use of TLI is that the procedure is not without significant side-effects. Severe leucopenia and throm-bocytopenia are common. Most candidates also suffer from severe nausea. These side-effects have, on occasion, been severe enough to warrant discontinuing the preconditioning regime. In addition, there is a significant risk of morbidity or mortality from infection occurring prior to transplantation. In this respect, patients in renal failure seem much more susceptible to the side-effects of TLI than those suffering from Hodgkin's disease. This apparent susceptibility has led to the TLI doses used in transplantation being reduced to between 2000 and 3000 rad instead of the 4000–5000 rad used for the treatment of Hodgkin's lymphoma.

There is undoubtedly a place for TLI in the treatment of graft rejection. It has proved particularly of value in preconditioning pre-sensitized individuals. Its ability to create an environment conducive to the production of chimeras must also hold out the promise of being able to establish donor-specific graft acceptance in the absence of any further immunosuppressive treatment.

PHARMACOLOGICAL IMMUNOSUPPRESSION

While donor-specific immunosuppression must ultimately be the goal for the treatment of the allograft recipient, the clinician faced with the urgency of treating fatal disease, often in the young, has been forced to turn to the less subtle approach of nonspecific immunosuppression in order to prevent graft rejection. Schwartz and Damashek[10] dis-covered that a short course of the antimetabolite, 6-mercaptopurine, would prevent rabbits from producing antibodies against heterologous proteins. 6-Mercaptopurine, given to dogs with renal allografts, showed that profound immunosuppression as assessed by graft sur-vival could be achieved with this agent[11], although the substance proved somewhat toxic, particularly to the liver. As a result of his initial observations with 6-mercaptopurine, Calne went on to study a number of purine and pyrimidine analogues of this drug. One of these analogues was azathioprine and Calne showed that it had a superior therapeutic index to 6-mercaptopurine for the immunosuppression of dogs with renal allografts[12]. Azathioprine was first used in clinical organ transplantation in 1962 by Murray[13] and his colleagues and has since proved to be one of the most valuable immunosuppressive drugs in organ transplantations. Although capable of acting as an antimetabolite for both adenine and hypoxanthine, the mode of action of azathioprine as an immunosuppressant has yet to be fully clarified. The side-effects of the drug can be significant, particularly depression of bone marrow cells. Some patients develop megaloblastic anaemia as a result of overdosing and the drug can also be hepatotoxic.

By 1963, azathioprine was being combined with corticosteroids[14] to prevent rejection in renal transplant recipients and this dual drug therapy has been the mainstay of immunosuppression in organ transplantation from that time. The dose of corticosteroids used in these initial transplant recipients was extremely high, some patients receiving as much as $5 \, mg \, kg^{-1} \, day^{-1}$. McGeown and her colleagues[15] demonstrated, however, that excellent results in renal transplantation could be obtained with relatively low doses of steroids and these studies led many groups to reappraise their dosage schedules. It is now customary to give steroids at an initial dose of $0.5–1 \, mg \, kg^{-1}$ and increase these doses during rejection episodes. The mechanism by which steroids exert an immunosuppressive effect is quite unclear but it is probably a combination of anti-inflammatory action, inhibition of cells migrating into the graft and thus coming in contact with antigen, and prevention of antigen-presenting cells from performing their function appropriately.

The use of corticosteroids in transplantation carries with it a significant risk of complications. Most of these can be attributed to the early post-transplant period when high doses of steroids were used and it is probable that most of the late complications seen in renal transplantation are a legacy of these early high doses of corticosteroids. Cushing's syndrome will persist only while the doses of steroids remain elevated and, as these doses are reduced, the hirsutism and moonfaces tend to become less marked. The effect of steroids on connective tissues can be seen in the skin which loses its elasticity and sometimes becomes extremely thin and frequently abraded and bruised. A significant percentage of patients treated with high doses of corticosteroids develop diabetes mellitus, the degree of glucose intolerance being closely related to the dosage of steroids given. The majority of such patients are able to discontinue insulin treatment and resume normal diets when prednisolone dosage is curtailed. A significant proportion of patients will develop pains in weight-bearing joints, particularly the hip. This complication usually starts 1–2 years post-transplant but may present at any time and total destruction of the femoral head with derangement of the joint can result. This avascular necrosis is well recognized in patients in long-term steroid treatment and can only be treated by total hip replacement. Visual blurring due to central posterior subcapsular cataracts occur in approximately 15% of steroid-treated transplant recipients. These are usually bilateral and must be extracted when they interfere significantly with central vision. Recurrent viral infections in the conjunctiva and cornea are also relatively common. It should be appreciated, however, that the risk of infection is always present in immunosuppressed patients and those treated with steroids remain exceedingly susceptible to certain virus infections, particularly those of the herpes group. Steroid therapy also carries with it a significant risk of peptic ulcers which may perforate or haemorrhage, requiring emergency surgery. The addition of salicylates to corticosteroid therapy appears to exacerbate the problem of gastric erosions and ulceration, probably by increasing the local erosive effect.

Although there is a marked variation from one centre to another, on average, the results of renal allografting using this dual therapy of azathioprine and steroids varied between 50% and 60% one-year graft survival. These figures have recently been considerably improved by the introduction into the immunosuppressive armamentarium of cyclosporin.

Cyclosporin

Cyclosporin was isolated from cultures of the fungal species, *Tolypocladium inflatum*, by biologists at Sandoz in Basel. It is a neutral, extremely hydrophobic, cyclical polypeptide composed of eleven amino acids, one of which is unique to the cyclosporins. Because of its extremely hydrophobic nature, the drug has to be dissolved in olive oil for its administration. The drug was first isolated as part of a search for biologically-produced antifungal agents. Although the compound proved to have only mild antifungal activity, it was discovered by Borel[16] to influence the immune system. On the basis of his initial observation, Borel suggested that the drug preferentially affected the activated, but not the resting, T cell at an early stage in the cell-activating process. Cyclosporin was first introduced into clinical transplantation by Calne *et al*. in Cambridge in 1978[17]. These clinical trials allowed a number of important conclusions on the use of this immunosuppressant to be made. First, cyclosporin is undoubtedly immunosuppressive for patients receiving cadaveric organ allografts. Second, the addition of cyclosporin to other immunosuppressive agents can produce drug cocktails which may be excessively immunosuppressive. Thus, the risk of life-threatening infection and the occurrence of Epstein–Barr virus-induced lymphomata may become unacceptably high; antilymphocyte globulins (ALG) have been particularly incriminated as dangerous when added to cyclosporin. Third, and perhaps most importantly, the drug is nephrotoxic to man at normal immunosuppressive doses, although this is not so in most animals. This last factor makes the drug difficult to manage in renal transplantation because the differential diagnosis between rejection and nephrotoxicity can be almost impossible to make and this may lead to unnecessary immunosuppression or delayed identification and treatment of rejection episodes.

The introduction of cyclosporin A into clinical transplantation by Calne and his colleagues[17] is one of the most important developments in recent years. The drug has been tested in a number of multicentre and single-centre trials for its efficacy in preventing kidney graft rejection. These trials established that immunosuppression with azathioprine and prednisolone invariably produced inferior results compared with cyclosporin[18]. Analyses from several large national databases of kidney transplants have shown that survival rates have improved with the introduction of cyclosporin by between 10 and 20% so that one-year graft survival in excess of 80% is now commonplace.

The use of cyclosporin A in combination with other immunosuppressive agents is, however, somewhat more controversial. Every combination of cyclosporin with prednisolone, azathioprine and ALG (and/or its monoclonal counterparts) has been advocated. In no case has an advantage over cyclosporin alone been demonstrated by appropriately-designed controlled trials. In contrast, several controlled trials have failed to demonstrate improved survival resulting from the addition of steroids to cyclosporin A immunosuppression.

While there is evidence that cyclosporin and steroids can produce a highly immunosuppressive cocktail, benefits accruing from prevention of rejection may well be counterbalanced by steroid complications and an increased incidence of infection. The current trend in clinical management is to use triple therapy in which cyclosporin, steroids and azathioprine are used in combination in relatively modest doses, thereby, in principle, reducing the side-effects of all three while maintaining a high degree of immunosuppression. This triple-therapy regimen is undoubtedly efficient, particularly in the reduction of the nephrotoxic side-effects of cyclosporin. However, several centres are now using low-dose ($6-8\,mg\,kg^{-1}$) cyclosporin therapy alone, apparently with equally good results.

Conversion from cyclosporin and prednisolone to azathioprine and prednisolone has been undertaken by a number of centres in order to reduce the financial burden of long-term cyclosporin therapy and for fear of the possible consequences of prolonged nephrotoxicity. After conversion at three months, Morris et al.[19] noticed a marked improvement in renal function, indicating that the nephrotoxic effect of cyclosporin was reversible at that time. However, conversion is followed by acute graft rejection in 30–50% of patients.

The clinical management of cyclosporin is greatly aided by the availability of blood or serum level measurements. These can be performed either by radioimmunoassay (RIA) or high-pressure liquid chromatography (HPLC). HPLC measurements provide a selective determination of the whole-drug concentrations only, while RIA, until recently, would also detect some metabolites. This problem with the RIA has now been resolved by the introduction of monoclonal antibody-based assays in which whole drug can be distinguished from metabolites. 40–60% of the drug concentration in the blood is bound to red cells while the remaining drug is associated with the lipoproteins. Because drug binding to cells is temperature dependent, the plasma must be separated from the erythrocytes at 37°C to obtain reproducible plasma levels. Thus, for convenience, most centres now determine the drug concentration of lysed whole blood since this approach avoids the temperature-dependent erythrocyte binding phenomenon. As cyclosporin is metabolized primarily by the liver and excreted by way of the bile, liver dysfunction can cause significant accumulation of both whole drug and metabolites, and management of cyclosporin in liver transplantation can be made much more difficult as a result of liver dysfunction.

Over the years, the recommended therapeutic window for whole blood or serum levels of cyclosporin has been steadily reducing so that most centres now aim their therapy at producing whole-blood trough levels in the 150–200 ng ml^{-1} range. Some centres are using even lower levels, apparently without hampering their success rate. Catabolism of the drug is accelerated by coincident administration of rifampicin or phenytoin by activating the cytochrome P450 pathway to increase the speed of degradation. Cyclosporin and prednisolone interact with each other by competing for this route of secretion. Concurrent therapy with aminoglycosides, trimethoprim, ketoconazole or amphotericin B also elevate cyclosporin blood levels and can result in increased nephrotoxicity[20].

Undoubtedly, the most significant side-effect of cyclosporin is its nephrotoxicity which is readily observed in humans but not in animals. This nephrotoxicity may become manifest in the early postoperative course or appear as a slow insidious decrease in renal function. The use of cyclosporin in patients whose kidney grafts do not diurese immediately postoperatively can result in very prolonged oliguria. In the Canadian multicentre trial, machine perfusion times of more than 24 hours and prolonged rewarming times longer than 45 minutes were shown to be specific risk factors for cyclosporin-treated patients. The risks involved were an increased incidence of primary non-function and a higher number of acute rejection episodes which required more frequent prednisone pulses for antirejection treatment. Cyclosporin also affects the liver, with serum bilirubin concentration increasing in direct relationship to the cyclosporin blood level. Serum transaminase levels are also occasionally elevated in a dose-dependent fashion. Hirsutism occurs in most patients taking cyclosporin; this is also dose dependent and will tend to disappear as the doses of cyclosporin are reduced. Tremor and paresthesia are fairly frequent complications of cyclosporin when used in high doses.

Monoclonal antibodies as immunosuppressants

It was suggested, at an early stage in the history of transplantation, that it may be advantageous to use a biological, rather than chemical, system to suppress the lymphocyte population. This was achieved, initially, by the relatively simple expedient of immunizing an animal with either lymphocytes or thymocytes, awaiting the development of antibodies to these cells, then purifying these antibodies from the serum of the animal. Such polyclonal antilymphocyte or anti-thymocyte sera have been raised in the rabbit, goat and horse.

Polyclonal ALG was first shown to have immunosuppressive properties by Woodruff and Anderson[21] who demonstrated delay in rejection of rat skin allografts in 1963. ALG was first used in clinical kidney transplantation in 1967[22] as a prophylactic agent, and as an effective means to reverse established rejection in 1970[23]. Subsequently, many trials have confirmed the efficacy of ALG as an immunosuppressive agent used both to prevent and to treat rejection. Such preparations are currently in routine use in clinical transplantation throughout the world; however, several important problems limit the efficacy of this approach to immunosuppression. First, polyclonal antibodies demonstrate considerable batch-to-batch variation in potency. Clearly, the precise composition of any one batch of ALG depends upon the response of the particular animal to immunization. Second, because the polyclonal preparation includes antibodies to a wide variety of antigens on the surface of lymphocytes, many of which are not exclusive to lymphocytes, antibodies are present which recognize cells other than lymphocytes. In practice, this lack of absolute specificity has proved less of a problem than might be expected and may, indeed, even be responsible for some of the beneficial properties of ALG. Third, because ALG contains such a wide variety of antibodies, the dose of immunoglobulin necessary to achieve a therapeutic effect is relatively large – typically 1 g or more. Regular infusions of foreign protein at such doses are likely to lead to 'serum sickness' in which antigen–antibody complexes form in the circulation. Finally, the production, purification and testing of these antibodies is complex and the cost of such preparations is relatively high.

With the technology to produce monoclonal antibodies[24] came the solution to many of these drawbacks to polyclonal antilymphocyte preparations. Monoclonal antibodies are produced by immunizing an animal (mouse or rat) with the appropriate antigenic stimulus (e.g. human lymphocytes), removing the spleen and fusing the cells of the spleen with those of a suitable mouse or rat myeloma. Such fusions produce a wide variety of cell lines containing a combination of genetic material. A proportion of these cell lines secrete antibodies which are specific for the immunizing antigens; the cell lines or clones grow in an uncontrolled fashion and continue to produce antibody. The cell lines produced in the fusion are then individually grown and the antibody produced by each is characterized.

Monoclonal antibody technology has the potential to produce almost limitless quantities of antibodies of a single specificity. The limitations of polyclonal preparations described above are thereby overcome. There is no batch-to-batch variation, the dose of antibody is, typically, 100-fold less, removing the risk of serum sickness, and there need be no reactivity with cells other than lymphocytes. The cost of monoclonal antibodies produced in ascites is considerable but it is possible to grow the clone in tissue culture – this is a considerably more efficient means of production of antibody in large quantities.

The fine specificity of monoclonal antibodies, however, raises new problems which were never encountered with polyclonal antibodies. Whereas polyclonal antibodies include a wide variety of specificities and isotypes, only a small proportion of which are pharmacologically active, in the case of monoclonal antibodies, the precise specificity which is pharmacologically active must be defined.

The development of antilymphocyte monoclonal antibodies as immunosuppressive agents has proceeded closely behind the definition of lymphocyte cell surface antigens. One of the major problems in considering monoclonal antibody therapy in immunosuppression is the large number of potentially useful antibodies available; it is not practical to test all these antibodies in formal clinical studies and animal models are not always available for the particular antibody and difficult to interpret.

When assessing an antilymphocyte monoclonal antibody for possible clinical use, there are several criteria which require consideration. The specificity of the antibody – the tissue distribution of the antigen recognized by the antibody – is clearly relevant to its *in vivo* properties. Unlike polyclonal antilymphocyte preparations, those monoclonal antilymphocyte antibodies which have been used for *in vivo* therapy in clinical transplantation recognize antigens which are expressed exclusively on the surface of peripheral blood mononuclear cells.

Depending upon the antigen recognized, monoclonal antibodies may recognize all peripheral blood lymphocytes (Campath-1)[25] or only T lymphocytes (OKT3)[26]. There are theoretical advantages in using a monoclonal antibody which is more effective in blocking or removing activated, as opposed to resting, T lymphocytes; for example, certain epitopes of the CD7 antigen are expressed more strongly after activation of the cell, and antibodies recognizing such epitopes are likely to exhibit 'activation bias'. Certain antigens are expressed on the surface of T lymphocytes only upon activation, and antibodies recognizing these antigens are, therefore, 'activation specific'. One example of an 'activation antigen' is the interleukin 2 receptor and a number of monoclonal antibodies have been described[27-29] which recognize this antigen. A major potential advantage of using such highly selective monoclonal antibodies as therapeutic agents is the ability to produce an immunosuppressive effect without unwanted effects on cells not involved in the rejection response. Theoretically, the use of such antibodies would leave intact the ability of the immune system to respond to other antigenic stimuli whenever treatment was stopped.

A second consideration is the effector mechanism. If an antibody recognizes a cell surface antigen which is essential for the normal function of the lymphocyte, it is likely to be effective merely by blocking that site. Similarly, if the binding of antibody to antigen leads to loss of the antigen from the cell surface, either by shedding or internalization (modulation), the antibody will have immunosuppressive properties even without the ability to lyse the cell. The CD3 antigen is one such 'functional' antigen; this is closely related to the T cell receptor and antibodies which block this site prevent normal activation of the cell in response to antigen. OKT3 is an antibody which recognizes the CD3 antigen; binding of OKT3 to its target leads to modulation of the receptor complex from the surface of the T cell and consequent loss of function of the cell. The reactions to the first dose of the antibody, which are characteristic of antibodies of this specificity, are due to activation of the T cells by the same binding process and consequent release of lymphokines. The ability of an antibody to block a functional antigen is a characteristic of the binding site of the antibody, the idiotypic region.

Alternatively, a monoclonal antibody may be effective as an immunosuppressive agent by cell killing rather than blocking cell function. An antibody which binds to a cell surface antigen but is not directly cytolytic may cause destruction of the cell by opsonization. However, more effective cell deletion results from either complement-mediated cytolysis, which requires the antibody to have the capability to bind human complement, or antibody-dependent cell-mediated cytotoxicity. The direct cytolytic activity of an antibody depends on the ability of the antibody to trigger host effector mechanisms and is a characteristic of the isotypic region of the antibody.

Pharmacokinetic considerations are also important in developing a monoclonal antibody for clinical use; it is necessary to devise a dosing schedule which achieves satisfactory serum and tissue levels of the antibody. This depends partly upon the size and frequency of dose but also upon the isotype of the antibody; the latter affects the rate of clearance of the antibody from the circulation and its ability to cross from the cardiovascular space to the extracellular space. For an antibody to exert maximal immunosuppressive effect, it is probably necessary for it to block or delete lymphocytes, not only in the cardiovascular space, but also within lymphoid tissue and the organ graft. The rate of clearance of an antibody from the circulation is also greatly increased by the presence of an antiglobulin response.

The development of an antiglobulin response has been demonstrated following administration of all clinically tested antibodies despite attempts to inhibit this with various agents, including cyclophosphamide and azathioprine. This response may be considered as two components; the anti-isotypic component, which recognizes the non-binding region of the antibody, and the anti-idiotypic component, which recognizes the binding region of the antibody. Because patients who make an antiglobulin response produce a combination of the two components, it is not yet entirely clear whether both components are clinically significant. It is likely that the presence of an anti-idiotypic response would lead to the monoclonal antibody becoming ineffective as the antiglobulin would compete with the lymphocytes for the binding sites of the antibodies. The significance of the anti-isotypic component is less clear, although binding to the antibody would presumably increase the rate of clearance of antibody.

Recent developments in monoclonal antibody therapy for solid-organ transplantation have been along two lines, the development of powerfully cytolytic antibodies and that of highly selective antibodies. In patients receiving a monoclonal antibody prophylactically, the principal concern is to avoid excessive immunosuppression and it is likely that the activation of selective antibodies will be of greatest benefit in providing immunosuppression without wide-ranging suppression of the immune response. In patients with established rejection, the principal concern is to block or delete lymphocytes as effectively as possible and it would seem reasonable that the most cytolytic antibody should be used in this context with less concern for the spectrum of activity. These two lines of development are not, however, mutually exclusive and there is no theoretical reason why a highly activation-selective antibody should not have extremely powerful cytolytic activity.

OKT3 has been used in clinical practice more widely than any other antibody and has been shown to be more effective in reversing rejection than high-dose steroids[30]. There is now increasing interest in the use of this antibody for prophylaxis[31]; it remains to be shown whether the effectiveness and side-effects of this antibody confer any advantage over polyclonal ALG in this context. Campath-1M has been shown to have a powerful immunosuppressive effect when used prophylactically[32]. The effectiveness of anti-IL2 receptor antibodies in prophylaxis has yet to be proven in controlled trials, although all centres which have tested such antibodies agree that the incidence of side-effects is minimal.

Future developments in the use of antilymphocyte monoclonal antibodies will depend upon increased knowledge of the nature of the rejection response and, in particular, the significance within it of various cell subsets. Highly effective deletion of the appropriate population of cells may lead to a much more specific approach to immunosuppression than has been possible previously and may, indeed, lead to the development of donor-specific tolerance. Human or 'humanized' antibodies are already under development and may prove superior to mouse- or rat-derived antibodies in a variety of ways. Such antibodies are likely to be more effective at interaction with host effector mechanisms; in addition, the propensity to induce an antiglobulin response should be less, allowing the course of antibody therapy to be either prolonged or repeated.

REFERENCES

1. Lindahl, K. E. and Wilson, D. B. (1977). Histocompatibility antigen-activated T lymphocytes. Estimates of the frequency and specificity of precursors. *J. Exp. Med.*, **145**, 508
2. Zinkernagel, R. M. and Doherty, P. C. (1974). Restriction of in vitro T cell mediated cytotoxicity in lymphocyte choriomeningitis with a syngeneic or semi allogeneic system. *Nature (London)*, **248**, 701
3. Matzinger, P. (1981). A one receptor view of T cell behaviour. *Nature (London)*, **292**, 497
4. Dallman, M. J. and Mason, D. W. (1982). Role of thymus derived and thymus independent cells in murine skin allograft rejection. *Transplantation*, **33**, 221
5. Hamburger, J., Vagsse, J. and Crosnier, J. (1962). Renal homotransplantation in man after radiation of the recipient. *Am. J. Med.*, **32**, 854
6. Slavin, S., Strober, S., Fuks, Z. and Kaplon, H. S. (1976). Long term survival of skin allografts in mice treated with total lymphoid irradiations. *Science*, **193**, 1252
7. Fuks, Z., Strober, S. and Bobrove, A. M. (1976). Long term effects of radiation on T and B lymphocytes in peripheral blood of patients with Hodgkin's disease. *J. Clin. Invest.*, **58**, 803
8. Slavin, S., Kaplon, H. S. and Strober, S. (1976). Transplantation of allogeneic bone marrow without graft versus host disease using total lymphoid irradiation. *J. Exp. Med.*, **147**, 963
9. Najarion, J. S., Ferguson, R. M., Sutherland, D. E. L., Slavin, S., Kim, T., Kersey, J. and Simons, R. L. (1982). Fractionated total lymphoid irradiation as preparative immunosuppression in high risk renal transplantation. *Ann. Surg.*, **196**, 442
10. Schwartz, R. and Damashek, W. (1959). Drug induced tolerance. *Nature (London)*, **183**, 1682
11. Calne, R. Y. (1960). The rejection of renal homografts inhibition in dogs by 6-mercaptopurine. *Lancet*, **1**, 417
12. Calne, R. Y. and Murray, J. E. (1961). Inhibition of the rejection of renal homografts in dogs with B20–322. *Surg. Forum*, **12**, 118
13. Murray, J. E., Merill, J. P., Harrison, J. H., Wilson, R. E. and Dammin, G. J. (1963). Prolonged survival of human kidney homografts by immunosuppressive drug therapy. *N. Engl. J. Med.*, **268**, 1315
14. Goodwin, W. E., Kaufman, J. J., Mimms, M. M., Turner, R. D., Glassock, K. R., Goldman, R. and Maxwell, M. M. (1963). Human renal transplantation clinical experiences with six cases of renal homotransplantation. *J. Urol.*, **89**, 13
15. McGeown, M. G., Douglas, J. E., Brown, M. D., Donaldson, R. A. and Hill, C. M. (1980). Advantages of low dose steroids from the day after transplantation. *Transplantation*, **29**, 287
16. Borel, J. F. (1976). Comparative study of in vitro and in vivo drug effects on cell mediated cytotoxicity. *Immunology*, **31**, 631

17. Calne, R. Y., White, D. J. G., Rolles, K., Thiru, S., Evans, D. B., McMaster, P. and Dunn, D. C. (1979). Cyclosporin A initially as the only immunosuppressant in 34 recipients of cadaveric organs: 32 kidneys, 2 pancreases and 2 livers. *Lancet*, **2,** 1033

18. Multi-author (1982). European multicentre trial. Cyclosporin A as sole immunosuppressive agent in recipients of kidneys from cadaver donors. *Lancet*, **2,** 57

19. Morris, P. J., French, M. F., Ting, A., Frostick, S. and Hunniset, A. (1982). A controlled trial of cyclosporin A in renal transplantation. In White, D. J. G. (ed.) *Cyclosporin A*, p. 355. (Amsterdam: Elsevier Biomedical)

20. Borel, J. F. (ed.) (1985). *Cyclosporin*. (Basel: Karger)

21. Woodruff, M. F. A. and Anderson, N. A. (1963). Effect of lymphocyte depletion by thoracic duct fistula and administration of anti-lymphocyte serum on the survival of skin homografts in rats. *Nature (London)*, **200,** 702

22. Starzl, T. E., Marchioro, T. L., Porter, K. A., Iwasaki, Y. and Cerilli, G. J. (1967). The use of heterologous antilymphoid agents in canine renal and liver homotransplantation and in human renal homotransplantation. *Surg. Gynecol. Obstet.* 301–318

23. Mee, A. D. and Evans, D. B. (1970). Antilymphocyte-serum preparations in treatment on renal-allograft rejection. *Lancet*, **2,** 16

24. Kohler, G. and Milstein, C. (1975). Continuous cultures of fused cells secreting antibody of predefined specificity. *Nature (London)*, **256,** 495

25. Hale, G., Bright, S., Chumbley, G. *et al.* (1983). Removal of T cells from bone marrow for transplantation: a monoclonal antilymphocyte antibody that fixes human complement. *Blood*, **62,** 873–882

26. Kung, P. C., Goldstein, G., Reinherz, E. L. and Schlossman, S. F. (1979). Monoclonal antibodies defining distinctive human T cell surface antigens. *Science*, **206,** 347–349

27. Tighe, H. P., Friend, P. J., Collier, St J. *et al.* (1988). Delayed allograft rejection in primates treated with anti-IL2 receptor monoclonal antibody Campath-6. *Transplantation*, **45,** 226–228

28. Shapiro, M. E., Kirkman, R. L., Reed, M. H. *et al.* (1987). Monoclonal anti-IL2 receptor antibody in primate renal transplantation. *Transplant. Proc.*, **19,** 594–598

29. Soulillou, J. P., Le Mauff, B., Olive, D. *et al.* (1987). Prevention of rejection of kidney transplants by monoclonal antibody directed against interleukin-2. *Lancet*, **2,** 1339 1342

30. Ortho Multicenter Transplant Study Group (1985). A randomized clinical trial of OKT3 monoclonal antibody for acute rejection of cadaveric renal transplants. *N. Engl. J. Med.*, **313,** 337–342

31. Debure, A., Chkoff, N., Chatenoud, L. *et al.* (1988). One month prophylactic use of OKT3 in cadaver kidney transplant recipients. *Transplantation*, **45,** 546–553

32. Friend, P. J., Calne, R. Y., Hale, G., Waldmann, H. *et al.* (1987). Prophylactic use of an antilymphocyte monoclonal antibody following renal transplantation – a randomised controlled trial. *Transplant. Proc.*, **19,** 1898–1900

INDEX